Cardiac Transplantation

Jeffrey D. Hosenpud   Adnan Cobanoglu
Douglas J. Norman   Albert Starr
Editors

Cardiac Transplantation

A Manual for
Health Care Professionals

Springer-Verlag New York Berlin Heidelberg
London Paris Tokyo Hong Kong Barcelona

JEFFREY D. HOSENPUD, M.D., Associate Professor of Medicine/Cardiology, Head, Cardiac Transplant Medicine, Oregon Health Sciences University, Portland, Oregon 97201, USA

ADNAN COBANOGLU, M.D., Professor of Surgery and Chief, Cardiopulmonary Surgery, Director, Heart Transplantation Program, Oregon Health Sciences University, Portland, Oregon 97201, USA

DOUGLAS J. NORMAN, M.D., Professor of Medicine, Director, Transplantation and Immunogenetics Laboratory, Director, Medical Transplantation Program, Oregon Health Sciences University, Portland, Oregon 97201, USA

ALBERT STARR, M.D., Professor of Surgery, Oregon Health Sciences University, Portland, Oregon 97201, USA

With 65 illustrations in 72 parts
Library of Congress Cataloging-in-Publication Data
Cardiac transplantation : a manual for health care professionals /
    J.D. Hosenpud . . . [et al.], editors,
        p.   cm.
    Includes bibliographical references.
    Includes index.
    ISBN 0-387-97304-4 (alk. paper)
    1. Heart—Transplantation—Handbooks, manuals, etc.   I. Hosenpud,
J. D. (Jeffrey D.)
    [DNLM: 1. Heart Transplantation.   WG 169 C2673]
RD598.35.T7C35   1990
617.4'120592—dc20
DNLM/DLC
for Library of Congress   90-9750

Printed on acid-free paper

Typeset by David E. Seham Associates, Inc., Metuchen, NJ.
Printed and bound by Edwards Brothers, Inc., Ann Arbor, MI.
Printed in the United States of America.

9 8 7 6 5 4 3 2 1

ISBN 0-387-97304-4 Springer-Verlag New York Berlin Heidelberg
ISBN 3-540-97304-4 Springer-Verlag Berlin Heidelberg New York

Preface

Over the past ten years, cardiac transplantation has evolved from an experimental procedure performed in a handful of university centers to a viable therapeutic modality now performed in more than 150 centers worldwide. The complexity of the procedure, the changing immunosuppressive regimes, and the follow-up care have necessitated a multidisciplinary approach involving a variety of medical, nursing, and social sciences specialties and subspecialties. In addition, health care trainees and referring physicians are increasingly becoming involved in the care of the cardiac transplant recipient. This book does not attempt to be a comprehensive treatise on cardiac transplantation; rather, we hope that it will serve as a manual and guideline for all health professionals involved in cardiac transplantation.

JEFFREY D. HOSENPUD, M.D.

Contents

Appendices

Contributors

ADNAN COBANOGLU, M.D.   Professor of Surgery and Chief, Cardiopulmonary Surgery, Director, Heart Transplantation Program, Oregon Health Sciences University, Portland, Oregon 97201, USA

JEFFREY D. HOSENPUD, M.D.   Associate Professor of Medicine/Cardiology, Head, Cardiac Transplant Medicine, Oregon Health Sciences University, Portland, Oregon 97201, USA

MARIAN C. LIMACHER, M.D.
Assistant Professor of Medicine, Transplant Cardiologist, University of Florida Medical Center, Gainesville, Florida 32610, USA

ROBERT A. MARICLE, M.D.   Associate Professor of Psychiatry, Director, Psychiatric Consultation and Liaison Service, Oregon Health Sciences University, Portland, Oregon 97201, USA

MARK J. MORTON, M.D.   Associate Professor of Medicine/Cardiology, Director, Catheterization Laboratory, Oregon Health Sciences University, Portland, Oregon 97201, USA

DOUGLAS J. NORMAN, M.D.   Professor of Medicine, Director, Transplantation and Immunogenetics Laboratory, Director, Medical Transplantation Program, Oregon Health Sciences University, Portland, Oregon 97201, USA

JOHN B. O'CONNELL, M.D.   Associate Professor of Medicine, Medical Director, UTAH Cardiac Transplant Program, University of Utah Medical Center, Salt Lake City, Utah 84132, USA

GEORGE A. PANTELY, M.D.   Associate Professor of Medicine, Oregon Health Sciences University, Portland, Oregon 97201, USA

D. GLENN PENNINGTON, M.D.   Professor of Surgery, St. Louis University Medical Center, Director, Heart Replacement Services, St. Louis, Missouri 63110, USA

JUDITH RAY, M.D.   Assistant Professor of Pathology, Oregon Health Sciences University, Portland, Oregon 97201, USA

DANIEL R. SALOMON, M.D.   Associate Professor of Medicine, Medical Director, Kidney and Heart Transplant Programs, University of Florida Medical Center, Gainesville, Florida 32610, USA

ALBERT STARR, M.D.   Professor of Surgery, Oregon Health Sciences University, Portland, Oregon 97201, USA

LYNNE WARNER STEVENSON, M.D.   Assistant Professor of Cardiology, UCLA School of Medicine, Director, Cardiomyopathy Center and Transplant Clinic, UCLA Center for the Health Sciences, Los Angeles, California 90024, USA

JEFFREY SWANSON, M.D.   Assistant Professor of Surgery, Oregon Health Sciences University, Portland, Oregon 97201, USA

MARC T. SWARTZ, B.A.   Director, Circulatory Support, Saint Louis University Medical Center, Saint Louis, Missouri 63110, USA

1
Cardiac Transplantation: An Overview

JEFFREY D. HOSENPUD AND ALBERT STARR

Cardiac transplantation has evolved from a highly experimental procedure to an accepted modality for the treatment of end-stage cardiac disease in slightly more than 20 years. In just the past 8 years the number
of hospitals performing cardiac transplantation has increased from 14 to
173 centers worldwide (Fig. 1.1), with the number of operations increasing from 92 to approximately 2500 in 1988 (Fig. 1.2). The obvious success
of cardiac transplantation can be attributed to substantial improvements
in a variety of areas, including preoperative management of congestive
heart failure, surgical techniques, donor management and organ preservation, prevention and treatment of rejection, and early and aggressive management of medical complications after transplantation. One-year survival has increased from around 70% to more than 85% in just the past 5
years, and long-term survival is now a realizable goal.[1] This chapter will
review the history of cardiac transplantation, its current successes and
limitations, and the evolution of the multidisciplinary approach to cardiac
transplantation.

Historical Perspective

Carrell and Guthrie[2] reported the first experience of transplanting the
heart in 1905. The operation consisted of anastomosing the great vessels,
cavae, and pulmonary vein of a smaller dog heart on to the carotid artery
and jugular vein of a larger dog. The circulation was subsequently maintained for approximately 90 min. Mann and colleagues[3] maintained allograft function for several days by using systemic anticoagulation and providing oxygenated blood to the donor coronary tree. Because of this
prolonged survival (8 days in the longest experiment), this group first recognized cardiac allograft rejection manifest clinically by ventricular fibrillation and pathologically by myocardial edema, necrosis, and an extensive myocardial mixed cellular infiltrate. Sinitsyn in 1948 first described a
working heterotopic cardiac transplant model,[4,5] and Demikhov, working

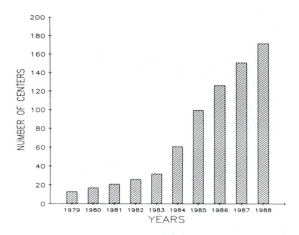

FIGURE 1.1. The number of centers performing cardiac transplantation has increased from 17 in 1980 to 173 in 1989. Reproduced from Heck et al. (1989),[1] with permission.

extensively through the 1940s, developed several methods, including an intrathoracic method for heterotopic cardiac transplantation.[4,5] Demikhov's longest surviving animal lasted 32 days, a feat even more remarkable considering the absence of myocardial preservation techniques and cardiopulmonary bypass.

With the advent of cardiopulmonary bypass, the stage was set for attempts to place the transplanted heart in the normal anatomic position.

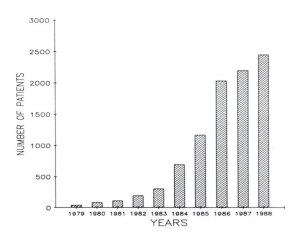

FIGURE 1.2. The number of cardiac transplant operations has increased almost exponentially in the 1980s, but the rate of increase has lessened over the past 2 years, and may be reaching a plateau. Reproduced from Heck et al. (1989),[1] with permission.

Berman and Goldberg[6,7] first noted that by preserving a cuff of left atrium, one eliminated the need for individual anastomosis of the pulmonary veins. The biatrial cuff preservation technique developed subsequently by Lower and Shumway[6,8] remains essentially unchanged today. The first orthotopic cardiac transplant operation to be attempted in humans was reported by Hardy and colleagues in 1964 using a chimpanzee heart.[9] Although the operation was technically successful, the smaller heart failed from acute volume overload. The first homologous human orthotopic heart transplant operation was performed by Barnard in 1967.[10] The patient survived for 18 days but ultimately succumbed to pneumonia.

As surgical techniques continued to be perfected, it became clear that the primary limitation of cardiac transplantation would be the immunologic rather than technical barriers. As early as 1943, Gibson and Medawar demonstrated that allograft rejection was primarily a cell-mediated process.[11,12] Overcoming this process became a major focus for research to make organ transplantation clinically applicable. Hume and colleagues in 1955 first demonstrated that corticosteroids alone did not appear to enhance survival of renal allografts.[13] In contrast, Schwartz and Dameshek demonstrated in 1959 that the antimetabolite 6-mercaptopurine reduced the immunologic response to organ transplantation.[14] Reemtsma and colleagues in 1962 first demonstrated that antimetabolites, specifically amethopterin, improved survival in canine heart transplantation.[15] Subsequently, the combination of glucocorticoids and antimetabolites were demonstrated to have complementary effects in organ transplantation,[16] and the combination of prednisone and azathioprine became the standard immunosuppressive regimen for organ transplantation until the early 1980s.

The next major advance in immunosuppression, the use of antilymphocyte antibodies, was proposed initially by Woodruff in 1960.[17] Ultimately, however, it required 12 years for the concept to find its way into experimental clinical practice in cardiac transplant patients, when the Stanford group reported improved survival and management of rejection using antilymphocyte globulin.[18]

The next major contribution to cardiac transplantation was diagnostic, not pharmacologic. Caves and colleagues at Stanford modified the Konno-Sakakibara transvenous bioptome and presented a series of patients who underwent surveillance endomyocardial biopsy after cardiac transplantation.[19] Using this technique, rejection could be detected at an early stage, before the development of clinical symptoms or signs. Moreover, the ability to diagnose the absence of rejection histologically enabled the investigators to reduce immunosuppression in a subset of patients, thereby reducing side effects. Surveillance endomyocardial biopsy has become the cornerstone of immunosuppression management and is the "gold standard" for the diagnosis of rejection.

The modern era of cardiac transplantation owes its current success largely to the discovery of cyclosporine A, a lipophilic cyclic polypeptide

TABLE 1.1. Surgical advances in heart transplantation.[a]

Date	Advance
1905	First heart transplantation in dogs (Carrell/Guthrie)
1933	Coronary perfusion in heart transplant in dogs (Mann)
1946	First thoracic heterotopic heart transplant in dogs (Demikhov)
1948	Sinitsyn-Marcus working donor heart
1959/60	Atrial cuff preservation (Berman, Goldbery and Lower, Shumway)
1963	First human lung transplantation (Hardy, Webb)
1964	First human heterologous heart transplantation (Hardy et al.)
1967	First human orthotopic homologous heart transplant (Barnard)

[a]Reproduced from Ontkean and Hosenpud (1989),[28] with permission.

from the fungus *Tolypocladium inflatum*.[20] This agent was found to be a potent immunosuppressive agent and was used initially in clinical trials for graft-versus-host disease,[21] and subsequently introduced in 1981 in heart transplantation, again by the Stanford group. Clinical trials with cyclosporine clearly demonstrated its superiority over traditional prednisone-azathioprine immunosuppression in cardiac transplantation,[22] and is now the mainstay of most transplant protocols. The remarkable success of this agent has prompted the search for similar compounds with the goals being greater specificity and efficacy and reduced side effects. One such agent, FK-506, is currently under active investigation in the animal laboratory,[23] but has only seen limited and thus far preliminary use in patients.[24]

In the past few years the direct application of molecular and cellular biologic techniques to medicine have produced major advances in transplantation. Using the hybridoma technique, first introduced by Kohler and Milstein,[25] a completely new class of agents, monoclonal antibodies, have been developed. The first to be released for clinical use in transplantation was OKT3, a monoclonal antibody directed against the T-cell CD3 surface molecule. The binding of this antibody after initially activating the T cell ultimately renders it incapable of responding to presented antigen.[26] OKT3 has been demonstrated to be a powerful immunosuppressant and is frequently successful in reversing rejection when all other methods of rejection therapy have failed.[27] Attempts to refine immunotherapy further by developing monoclonal antibodies directed against only activated lymphocytes, and hybrid monoclonal antibodies coupled to cytotoxins, are currently under active investigation. Advances in surgical techniques and immunosuppression are summarized in Tables 1.1 and 1.2, respectively.[28]

Current State of Cardiac Transplantation

Owing in large part to the perseverance and ultimate successes of the Stanford group and other pioneers in the field, cardiac transplantation has emerged as an accepted modality for the treatment of heart failure.

TABLE 1.2. Advances in immunosuppression in heart transplantation.[a]

Date	Advance
1955	ACTH and cortisone used in renal transplantation
1960	6-mercaptopurine used in canine heart transplantation
1963	Azathioprine enhances renal transplant survival in humans
1965	Antilymphocyte treatment for renal transplant acute rejection
1971	Antilymphocyte treatment for heart transplant acute rejection
1978	Discovery of cyclosporine and introduction in renal transplant
1981	Monoclonal antibody introduction in renal transplant rejection
1981	Introduction of cyclosporine in heart transplantation
1985	Monoclonal antibody OKT3 used in heart transplantation

[a]Reproduced from Ontkean and Hosenpud (1989),[28] with permission.

Although the centralization of this procedure for the initial 15 years is largely responsible for this success, the expansion into multiple centers in the 1980s has had the advantage of infusing new ideas and approaches to these patients and ultimately improvement in quality and quantity of life. Figure 1.3 demonstrates the four-year actuarial survival of the first 89 patients transplanted at Oregon Health Sciences University. This reported survival is essentially identical to that reached by most major transplant centers in the United States and Europe.[1] Because of these results, recipient criteria have been expanded gradually to include older aged patients (in most centers up to age 60 years and in some up to age 65 years), diabetic patients without end-organ damage, and even some patients with prior malignancies if now considered cured. In addition to the substantial improvement in survival after cardiac transplantation, the quality of survival in general is excellent. In a study of 100 recipients,

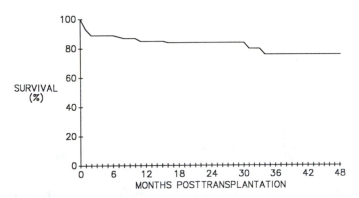

FIGURE 1.3. Survival after cardiac transplantation at Oregon Health Sciences University is 86% at 1 year and 76% at 4 years. This is not significantly different from survival reported by the Registry of the International Society for Heart Transplantation.[1]

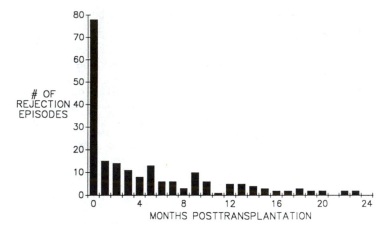

FIGURE 1.4. Acute rejection occurs most frequently in the first months after cardiac transplantation, but continues to occur throughout the posttransplant period.

quality of life was judged to be either excellent or very good in 67% of the patients queried.[29]

The major problems and most frequent causes of death early posttransplantation continue to be acute rejection and infection, and although the incidence of these complications decreases substantially with time, they continue to be potential problems even late after cardiac transplantation (Figs. 1.4, 1.5). The multiple side effects of the immunosuppressive

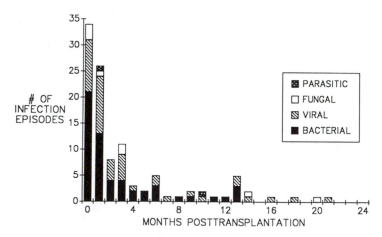

FIGURE 1.5. Infection, like rejection, occurs most frequently early after cardiac transplantation, and is probably related to the increased need for immunosuppression early on. Bacterial and viral infections (CMV) are most common, but fungal and parasitic infections also add significant morbidity.

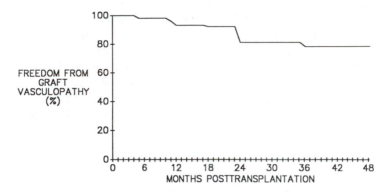

FIGURE 1.6. The incidence of coronary vasculopathy is 7% at 1 year and 19% at 2 years in the Oregon program. This is not dissimilar to the incidence of this problem reported in the literature,[30] and is responsible for a significant proportion of the late morbidity and mortality that follows cardiac transplantation.

agents, including bone disease, malignancy, hypertension, renal dysfunction, obesity, and others, contribute to morbidity in a substantial number of patients.

The complication that impacts long-term survival most importantly is a peculiar form of accelerated vasculopathy superficially similar to coronary atherosclerosis, which occurs in the allograft at a rate of 10% to 15% per year.[30] The overall prevalence of this lesion is as high as 45% of all recipients by 5 years. Figure 1.6 demonstrates the slightly (but probably not significantly) lower prevalence of this vasculopathy at Oregon Health Sciences University. The process is a diffuse one, and involves the entire allograft coronary tree resulting in occlusion of distal vessels. Because of its rapid onset and in some studies association with acute rejection,[31] it is felt to be immunologic in nature. Recent studies have suggested an association with cytomegalovirus.[32] However, the specific mechanisms responsible for this vasculopathy are yet to be discovered. Until this serious problem can be resolved, truly long-term survival for a large portion of patients after cardiac transplantation will not be realized. It is precisely for this reason that cardiac transplantation must be reserved for truly end-stage cardiac disease for which there is no alternative treatment.

Organization of the Cardiac Transplant Team

The evolving complexity of the field of transplantation is responsible for another change in the approach to cardiac transplantation: from that of a surgical subspecialty to that of a multidisciplinary one. In addition to the cardiac transplant surgeon, the team now comprises cardiologists, immunologists, psychiatrists, social workers, and specially trained nurses. This multidisciplinary approach is now also recognized by the United Network for Organ Sharing, and all of these disciplines must be in place in order for a cardiac transplant program to be certified. Although the specific responsibilities of these individuals may vary somewhat from institution to institution, the basic roles are becoming increasingly defined. The following recommended structure is based on the Cardiac Transplant Program at Oregon Health Sciences University.

Cardiac Transplant Surgeon

The responsibilities of the cardiac transplant surgeon fall into two major categories involving the donor and the recipient. The surgeon is responsible for the evaluation and subsequent management of the donor who has been identified as a possible heart donor, and the ultimate acceptance and retrieval of the donor heart. The cardiac transplant surgeon is ultimately responsible for the initial success of the cardiac transplant operation; therefore, he must have control over the "raw materials" required for that success.

The cardiac transplant surgeon is responsible for multiple phases of recipient care. First, after initial evaluation of the recipient, it is the surgeon's responsibility to identify active issues that may directly impact on surgical success (prior operation, internal mammary bypass grafts, anticoagulation, nutritional status, etc.). The surgeon should also be prepared to consider surgical alternatives to cardiac transplantation if indicated. Once the recipient is admitted to the hospital for cardiac transplantation, the transplant surgeon is then responsible for the immediate preoperative, operative, and early postoperative in-patient surgical care. Finally, the cardiac transplant surgeon is responsible for surgical complications that arise at any time after cardiac transplantation. A hospital that has a large cardiovascular and cardiac surgical service (500 open heart cases per year) and the added burden of cardiac transplantation should not require the addition of new cardiac surgical staff, given the comparatively low volume of transplantations. Smaller programs should have available at least three cardiac surgeons competent in cardiac transplantation to ensure the availability of at least two (donor team and recipient team) surgeons at all times.

Cardiac Transplant Physician/Cardiologist

The cardiac transplant physician is a cardiologist who specializes in the care of end-stage heart disease and transplantation medicine. The responsibilities of the transplant cardiologist begin at the initial referral of a potential cardiac transplant recipient. This individual should have extensive knowledge of the natural history of end-stage cardiac disease and where a given patient fits on this natural history curve; this individual therefore determines whether and when it is appropriate to consider a patient referred for cardiac transplantation. It is then this individual's responsibility for the initial evaluation and care of the candidate. After the evaluation and acceptance of the recipient as a candidate for cardiac transplantation by the transplant committee, the transplant cardiologist is responsible for maintaining the stability of the candidate, determining need for hospitalization, and with the transplant surgeon is responsible for the decision of whether a candidate requires additional support beyond medical management (i.e., ventricular assistance). In addition, this individual is responsible for determining a given patient's medical priority, based on standard criteria.

After cardiac transplantation, the transplant cardiologist follows the patient with the transplant surgeon within the early postoperative period, assisting in the interpretation of cardiovascular signs, symptoms, and diagnostic studies. This individual is usually responsible for performing surveillance endomyocardial biopsies and diagnostic catheterization, and with the assistance of the transplant immunologist (may be the same person) is responsible for directing both maintenance and rescue immunosuppression. Over the longer term, the transplant cardiologist is responsible for managing the patient in the out-patient setting in all aspects of the patient's care. In contrast to the requirements for cardiac surgical staff, the cardiac transplant cardiologist essentially becomes the primary care physician. Because of the successful outcomes leading to longer term survival and the intensive follow-up required, individuals dedicated to transplantation are required. For most medium-volume programs a minimum of two cardiac transplant cardiologists are necessary to accomplish these tasks.

Transplant Immunologist

The transplant immunologist is frequently a resource for all of the organ transplant programs within an institution. Often this individual is also responsible for the administration of the immunology and tissue typing laboratory. The responsibility of this individual is to assist in the immunologic monitoring of patients before and after transplantation, to identify patients at high risk for early immunologic complications (i.e., the highly sensitized individual), and to recommend and facilitate pretransplant screening and posttransplant specialized immunologic therapy. In addition, this individual is responsible for assisting in the design and monitoring of immunosuppression protocols, laboratory monitoring of specific immunosuppression such as monoclonal antibody therapy, and to assist in more unusual forms of therapy (i.e., plasmaphoresis). Finally, this individual should serve as a resource for the early experience with new or experimental immunosuppressive agents, because frequently this individual, being involved with multiple transplant programs, will have a greater overall experience with these agents.

Cardiac Transplant Psychiatrist

As with the other individuals involved, the transplant psychiatrist has responsibilities both before and after cardiac transplantation. This individual will evaluate prospective cardiac transplant recipient candidates specifically to investigate past behaviors that may impact pre- and postoperative care. The evaluation is in almost all circumstances used not to exclude individuals from cardiac transplantation (although in extreme cases this has occurred), but to identify tendencies in a given individual that can either be modified using preventative measures, or, if not, can allow the team to take a modified approach to this individual in an attempt to minimize conflicts or problems.

Given the individual and family stresses that are present throughout the transplant experience, the transplant psychiatrist is a resource for counseling. In addition, it is important for this individual to be well versed not only in psychiatric clinical pharmacology, but cardiovascular and specifically cardiac transplant physiology and pharmacology, so that effective pharmacologic therapy can be instituted where needed.

Cardiac Transplant Social Worker

Cardiac transplantation requires a substantial commitment from the patient and the patient's family. Initially it is the transplant social worker's responsibility to document the presence of family and/or other nonfamily support and commitment to the transplantation. In addition, as most transplant programs require that the patient be within close proximity, many patients and their families must move to the city containing the transplant center. This can frequently create psychological and financial stresses. It is the responsibility of the transplant social worker to assist in these relocations and their accompanying problems.

In the United States, most (if not all) transplant centers require that the patient have financial support for the expenses incurred for the transplant operation. Most patients undergoing cardiac transplantation have third-party coverage (private insurance carriers), some transplants are funded by Medicare, and in some states Medicaid. In those individuals not having obvious funding, the transplant social worker will investigate all options for transplant funding. In addition, after cardiac transplantation, the patient's status with regard to disability, insurability, and ongoing financial obligations may require preemptive planning to make every effort to ensure that lapses in funding, which can be financially devastating to the patient and patient's family, do not occur.

Finally, the transplant social worker, in conjunction with the transplant psychiatrist, is a resource for patient and family counseling.

Cardiac Transplant Nurse Coordinator

The cardiac transplant nurse coordinator probably has the most important and demanding role of all members of the cardiac transplant team. The transplant coordinator is responsible for the coordination of all aspects of the patient's care pre-, peri-, and postoperatively. The responsibilities can be grouped into two main categories: patient care and teaching. The coordinators direct the pretransplant evaluation and participate in post-transplant care and scheduling of follow-up visits and diagnostic studies. They are responsible for screening and identifying patient clinical and laboratory problems in both the in-patient and out-patient settings, and referring these to the physician caring for the patient. The transplant coordinator is usually the cardiac transplant recipient's primary contact when physical or psychological problems develop. Therefore, a substantial amount of patient counseling is also required.

The transplant coordinator has a primary role in education at all levels. This includes the education of the patient and family with regard to all aspects of cardiac transplantation, medications and side effects, and patient responsibilities. In addition, the coordinator is responsible for the education of all hospital nursing and ancillary care. Finally, there is a substantial demand on these individuals to provide community outreach and education, to both the medical and lay public. The experience at Oregon Health Sciences University suggests an approximate ratio of one transplant coordinator for every 25 to 30 transplant recipients being followed by a given program.

Conclusions

The current state of cardiac transplantation, to be fully outlined in the following chapters, owes its success to half a century of investigative and clinical work. It has evolved over the past 20 years from a highly experimental curiosity to almost routine, albeit intensive, care for end-stage cardiac disease. Cardiac transplantation is now a multidisciplinary team effort and requires a substantial institutional resource commitment to ensure its success. Despite that, the outcome measured both in quality and quantity of patient survival and the cost effectiveness of the procedure has continued to improve over the past decade, and should continue to improve over the next.

References

1. Heck CF, Shumway SJ, Kaye MP. The Registry of the International Society of Heart Transplantation. Sixth official report—1989. *J Heart Transplant.* 1989;8:271–276.
2. Carrell A, Guthrie CC. The transplantation of veins and organs. *Am Med.* 1905;10:1101–1102.

3. Mann FC, Priestley JT, Markowitz J. Transplantation of the mammalian heart. *Arch Surg.* 1933;26:219–224.
4. Cooper KC, Lanza RP. Experimental development and early clinical experience. In: Cooper KC, Lanza RP, eds. *Heart Transplantation*. MTP Press Ltd; 1984:1–14.
5. Myerowitz PD. The history of heart transplantation. In: Myerowitz PD, ed. *Heart Transplantation*. Mt. Kisco, NY: Futura Publishing Co Inc; 1987:1–17.
6. Lower RR, Shumway NE. Studies on orthotopic homotransplantation of the canine heart. *Surg Forum.* 1960;11:18–19.
7. Shumway NE, Lower RR. Special problems in transplantation of the heart. *Ann NY Acad Sci.* 1964;120:773–777.
8. Lower RR, Stoferr RC, Shumway NE. Homovital transplantation of the heart. *J Thorac Cardiovasc Surg.* 1961;41:196–204.
9. Hardy JD, Webb WR, Dalton ML, et al. Heart transplantation in man: developmental studies and report of a case. *JAMA.* 1964;88:1132–1140.
10. Barnard CN: A human cardiac transplant: an interim report of a successful operation performed at Groote Schuur Hospital, Cape Town. *S Afr Med J.* 1967;41:1271.
11. Gibson T, Medawar PB. The fate of skin homografts in man. *J Anat.* 1942–43;77:299–310.
12. Medawar PB. A second study of the behavior and fate of skin homografts in rabbits. *J Anat.* 1945;79:157–176.
13. Hume DM, Merrill JP, Miller BF, et al. Experiences with renal homotransplantation in the human: report in nine cases. *J Clin Invest.* 1955;34:327–382.
14. Schwartz R, Dameshek W. Drug-induced immunologic tolerance. *Nature.* 1959;183:1682–1683.
15. Reemtsma K, Williamson WE, Inglesias F, et al. Studies in homologous canine heart transplantation: prolongation of survival with a folic acid antagonist. *Surgery.* 1962;52:127–133.
16. Murray JE, Merril JP, Harrison JH, et al. Prolonged survival of human kidney homografts by immunosuppressive drug therapy. *N Engl J Med.* 1963;268:1315–1323.
17. Woodruff MF. The effect of various experimental procedures on the behaviour of homotransplants. In: Woodruff MFA, ed. *The Transplantation of Human Tissues & Organs*. New York, NY: Charles C Thomas Publisher; 1960:98–113.
18. Griepp RB, Stinson EB, Dong E, et al. Use of antithymocyte globulin in human heart transplantation. *Circulation.* 1972;45:I147–I153.
19. Caves PK, Stinson EB, Billingham ME, et al. Diagnosis of human cardiac allograft rejection by serial cardiac biopsy. *J Thorac Cardiovasc Surg.* 1973;66:461–466.
20. Borel JF, Feurer C, Magnee C, et al. Effects of the new antilymphocytic peptide cyclosporine A in animals. *Immunology.* 1977;32:1017–1025.
21. Calne RY, Thiru S, McMaster P, et al. Cyclosporine A in patients receiving renal allografts from cadaver donors. *Lancet.* 1978;23:1323–1331.
22. Oyer PE, Stinson EB, Jamieson SE, et al. Cyclosporine in cardiac transplantation, a $2\frac{1}{2}$ year follow-up. *Transplant Proc.* 1983;15:2546–2552.
23. Yokota K, Takishima T, Sato K, et al. Comparative studies of FK506 and cyclosporine in canine orthotopic hepatic allograft survival. *Transplant Proc.* 1989;21:0166–1068.

24. Starzl TE, Fung J, Venkataramman R, Todo S, Demetris AJ, Jain A. FK 506 for liver, kidney and pancreas transplantation. *Lancet*. 1989;2:1000–1004.
25. Kohler G, Milstein C. Continuous cultures of fused cells secreting antibody of predefined specificity. *Nature*. 1975;256:495–497.
26. Norman DJ. The clinical role of OKT3. *Transplant Immunol*. 1989;9:95–107.
27. Gilbert EM, Dewitt CW, Eiswirth CC, et al. Treatment of refractory cardiac allograft rejection with OKT3 monoclonal antibody. *Am J Med*. 1987;82:202–206.
28. Ontkean M, Hosenpud JD: Emergence of routine survival following orthotopic cardiac transplantation. *Heart Fail*. 1989;5(6):219–227.
29. Lough ME, Lindsey AM, Shinn JA, Stotts NA. Life satisfaction following heart transplantation. *J Heart Transplant*. 1985;4:446–449.
30. Billingham ME. Cardiac transplant atherosclerosis. *Transplant Proc*. 1987;19:19–25.
31. Narrod J, Kormos R, Armitage J, et al. Acute rejection and coronary artery disease in long term survivors of heart transplantation. *J Heart Transplant*. 1989;8:418–421.
32. Gratten MT, Moreno-Cabral CE, Starnes VA, et al. Cytomegalovirus infection is associated with cardiac allograft rejection and atherosclerosis. *JAMA*. 1989;261:3561–66.

2
Immunogenetics and Immunologic Mechanisms of Rejection

Douglas J. Norman

Basic Immunogenetics

The major histocompatibility complex (MHC) is a group of genes found in a region on the short arm of the sixth chromosome in man (Fig. 2.1).[1] This region codes for histocompatibility antigens that are known to be the strongest barriers to transplantation of organs from one human individual to another[2]; these antigens elicit strong immune responses when they are not matched. Experience in kidney allograft transplantation has demonstrated that matching for these antigens within families and between unrelated individuals (as in cadaveric kidney transplantation) significantly reduces the strength of the immune response and leads to superior graft survival.[3] This is also the case in bone marrow transplantation, wherein successful engraftment relies on both the absence of rejection and the absence of a graft-versus-host reaction. To achieve this, the histocompatibility antigen discrepancy must be minimal when donor cells scrutinize the recipient and when recipient cells scrutinize donor cells.[4] All vertebrate animals that have been studied, including rodents, dogs, lower primates, and swine, have a major histocompatibility complex. In man, the glycoprotein gene products of the major histocompatibility complex are known as human leukocyte antigens, or HLA.

In practice, identifying the HLA antigens of both the donor and recipient and choosing an optimal donor by matching for these before to transplantation can be accomplished in kidney and bone marrow transplantation. However, in liver, pancreas, and heart transplantation prospective matching has been impractical mainly because of the limited ischemia times allowable for successful outcomes. Despite the practical impediments to prospective HLA antigen typing and matching in cardiac transplantation, retrospective analyses have demonstrated that high-grade HLA antigen matches can be superior to poor matches.[5] In the future, if preservation techniques are improved and if intra- and interregional sharing agreements are established, it may be possible to share heart allografts

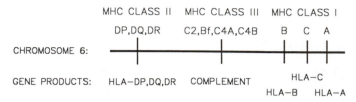

FIGURE 2.1. The schematic representation of the genes coding for the MHC found on the short arm of chromosome 6 in humans. Class I genes code for HLA-A, HLA-B, and HLA-C antigens. Class II genes code for HLA-DP, HLA-DQ, and HLA-DR. Class III genes code for several of the complement proteins.

on the basis of prospective typing and matching. Based on published literature this might improve overall heart allograft survival.[5]

Rather than for purposes of transplantation, the major histocompatibility antigens exist to facilitate the immune response elicited by an individual against foreign tissues and to recognize oneself.[6] The immune response is MHC-restricted; that is, important cells of the immune response see foreign antigens in the context of their own MHC antigens. In fact, upon processing by accessory or antigen presenting cells (e.g., macrophages), these foreign antigens are actually presented along with the major histocompatibility antigens to the immune cells.[7]

Each individual has two number six chromosomes and therefore two haplotypes for the MHC genes (Fig. 2.1). The genes coding for HLA antigens are co-dominant, resulting in equal expression of the gene products of each of the MHC genes on both chromosomes. The genes of the MHC have been divided into three classes.

Products of Class I genes consist of a 45,000-Dalton heavy chain. A noncovalently bound light chain known as beta-2 microglobulin is coded by genes on another chromosome. The heavy chain of Class I molecules extends through the cell membrane and into the cytoplasm, but most of the molecule is found on the exterior of the cell. The Class I molecules are known as HLA A, B, and C. One of the remarkable aspects of the major histocompatibility genes is their polymorphism. In other words, each gene has a number of different alleles. For example, more than 25 different HLA A antigens, 40 different HLA B antigens, and 15 different HLA C antigens have been identified.[8] Class I gene products are found on all nucleated cells in the body, including platelets, but are not found on mature red blood cells. Owing to their universal presence on transplanted organs, Class I antigens are the primary target of a host immune response.

Products of the Class II genes are an alpha and beta chain of approximately equal molecular weight, 45,000 Daltons, each penetrating the cell membrane and extending into the cytoplasm. However, as is the case with Class I antigens, Class II antigens are found predominantly on a

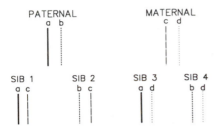

FIGURE 2.2. The inheritance of genes coding for MHC antigens follow mendelian inheritance patterns. As each parent has two haplotypes, there are four potential combinations of haplotypes in the progeny (excluding recombinations). Therefore, the chances that a sibling will be an identical HLA match with another sibling are 1 in 4 (25%). The likelihood of sharing at least one haplotype with another sibling is 1 in 2 (50%).

cell's surface. The best described Class II antigens are known as HLA DP, DQ, and DR. Class II genes are also polymorphic and have a number of different alleles. Defined HLA DR antigens include approximately 20, DP approximately 6, and DQ 8.[8] Class II antigens have a much more limited tissue distribution than Class I antigens. Class II antigens are found predominantly on antigen-presenting or accessory cells such as monocytes, macrophages, and dendritic cells as well as on B cells, sperm, and to a limited extent on venous endothelial cells, which also have the capability of antigen presentation. Activated cells of all types including endothelial cells express Class II molecules.

Products of the Class III genes include three important components of the complement system of proteins: C2, C4, and Bf.[9]

Inheritance of the HLA antigens follows standard mendelian genetics. Each chromosome contains one haplotype and therefore each person has two haplotypes. One haplotype is inherited from each parent. Twenty-five percent of siblings are matched for both haplotypes, 50% are matched for one haplotype, and another 25% are matched for zero haplotypes (Fig. 2.2).

Laboratory methods for identifying actual genes have been established.[10] However, for practical purposes, instead of identifying genes for tissue typing, laboratory techniques for identifying gene products are mainly being used. Tissue typing has been made relatively easy because all of the major histocompatibility gene products can be found on circulating leukocytes. Specific alloantisera defining Class I and Class II antigens have been obtained from multiparous women who make these antisera as a natural consequence of becoming pregnant on multiple occasions. Monoclonal antibodies that are capable of recognizing some of the HLA antigens have been manufactured and these also can be used for tissue typing. The basic ingredients for tissue typing assays are (1) alloantisera defining specific HLA antigens and (2) leukocytes, specifically T cells and B cells from an individual whose tissue type is desired.

The HLA antigens that are identified by allosera are know as "serologi-

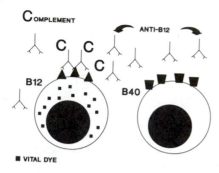

FIGURE 2.3. Complement-dependent antibody-mediated cytotoxicity. This microlymphocytotoxicity technique is the primary tool for tissue typing for HLA-A, B, C, and DR antigens, for screening for preformed antibodies to HLA antigens, and for performing the standard crossmatch. In the first instance, multiple tissue typing sera containing high titers of antibody against known HLA antigens are reacted against the patient's circulating lymphocytes (the unknown). In the second, the patient's serum (unknown) is reacted to a panel of lymphocytes containing a wide representation of known HLA antigens. In the third, the recipient's serum (unknown) is reacted with the donor's circulating lymphocytes (unknown). In all cases one is testing for specific anti-HLA antibody binding to lymphocytes, which in the presence of complement causes membrane rupture and allows the infusion of a vital dye (in most cases eosin). In this schematic, anti-HLA-B12 reacts against a lymphocyte with the B12 phenotype, but not against a lymphocyte with the B40 phenotype.

cally defined" HLA antigens and these include HLA A, B, and C, and DR and DQ (see Fig. 2.3). "Lymphocyte defined" antigens that are not serologically definable may also exist. These antigens are identified by mixing lymphocytes (see Fig. 2.4) from an individual with a panel of irradiated homozygous typing cells of known HLA Class II tissue types in a mixed lymphocyte culture.[11] Reactivity patterns are analyzed to determine the HLA "D" type. The "D" type of a patient is that of the one or more homozygous typing cells against which there is no reaction. If a patient is heterozygous (e.g., HLA D2, D3) for the "D" antigens, his cells will be nonreactive with two different cells on the panel.

The MHC is not the only histocompatibility complex; minor histocompatibility antigens coded for by genes in other regions of the human genome are also known to exist. For example, in the mouse, whose MHC is found on the 17th chromosome,[12] many minor histocompatibility genes have also been identified and are scattered throughout the mouse genome. Minor histocompatibility antigens are called minor because they elicit weak immune responses, but in the absence of recipient manipulation with immunosuppression they can stimulate organ graft rejection. However, rejection is less vigorous and requires a longer time to develop. Minor histocompatibility antigen differences between HLA identical siblings who share two HLA haplotypes accounts for the small incidence of graft loss in HLA identical kidney transplantation and also for the graft-versus-host disease and rejection encountered in bone marrow transplantation between HLA identical siblings.

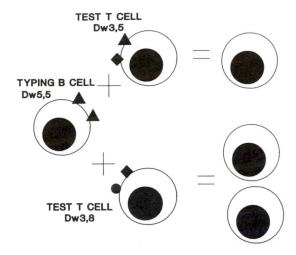

FIGURE 2.4. The mixed lymphocyte reaction is used for HLA-D typing. Irradiated typing B lymphocytes with known HLA phenotypes (in this case homozygous for HLA-Dw5) are reacted against T lymphoctyes of unknown phenotype. In the presence of lymphocytes with a shared phenotype (Test T cell Dw3, 5), no reaction occurs and the lymphocyte is not stimulated to proliferate. However, in the presence of lymphocytes with no shared D antigens (Test T cell Dw3,8), the test lymphocytes are stimulated to proliferate (usually measured by tritiated thymidine uptake).

Clinical Immunogenetics/Tissue Typing

Clinical immunogenetics, or tissue typing, is the application of the practical aspects of immunogenetics to clinical medicine. In organ transplantation this includes: (1) HLA typing of the donor and recipient, (2) measurement of anti-HLA antibodies in the recipient's serum by reacting the patient's serum with a panel of lymphocytes of known tissue type, a determination that will predict the chances of finding a compatible organ for a recipient, and (3) performing the final crossmatch between the donor and recipient, a test that determines if the recipient has antibodies that can react specifically with donor cells, a condition that can lead to hyperacute or accelerated rejection.[13]

The tissue type of the recipient can be obtained at any time before transplantation. The tissue type of the donor is obtained only at the time of transplantation because all donors for heart transplantation are cadaveric. The HLA A and B antigen types are determined by using peripheral blood lymphocytes from the donor or the recipient. The HLA DR tissue type is determined by using B lymphocytes because of the aforementioned tissue distribution of the Class II antigens. Concordance between laboratories for typing of the Class I antigens is now greater than 97%.

Concordance for typing the Class II antigens is only about 90%, owing to the more difficult procedure involved with typing of B cells and also because of the poorer overall quality of Class II typing reagents compared with Class I reagents. Some individuals are homozygous for one or more HLA antigen; for example, an HLA type may be HLA A1, B8, DR3, DR4 due to the homozygosity for A1 and B8. Individuals who are not homozygous for any of these antigens should have six identifiable antigens: two HLA A antigens, two HLA B antigens and two HLA DR antigens. Knowing the HLA type of the donor and the recipient in heart transplantation is useful mainly to establish retrospectively whether or not HLA matching is beneficial.

The Crossmatch

Occasionally prospective cardiac transplant patients develop anti-HLA antibodies as a result of transfusions, pregnancy, or prior transplants. These anti-HLA antibodies can cause immediate or accelerated graft loss if they are directed against donor HLA antigens.[13] There are now adequate numbers of reported cases of hyperacute rejection occurring because of preexistent antidonor antibodies to warrant a careful screening of patients for these antibodies during the recipient evaluation process. To accomplish this screening, a patient's serum is generally tested for its reactivity against a panel of lymphocytes (see Fig. 2.3). Most lymphocyte panels consist of cells from 48 to 60 individuals and are selected so that all of the known HLA antigen types are represented. If a panel is carefully selected, specific antigens can be identified against which the recipient may have antibodies.

The term "PRA" stands for panel reactive antibodies, and "percent PRA" refers to the percent of the panel with which an individual patient's serum reacts. As an example, if a patient's serum reacts with cells from 12 of the 48 individuals selected for a panel, the PRA would be 25%. Generally speaking, the percent PRA predicts the probability that a patient would be crossmatch-positive with any given donor. However, this is not always the case. Since approximately one-half of the North American Caucasian population carries the HLA A2 antigen,[14] a prospective heart transplant patient who has an anti-HLA A2 antibody predictably would be crossmatch-positive with one-half of the prospective cardiac donors. However, his serum might react with only a small percentage of the cells of individuals chosen for the lymphocyte panel because of a desire to create a panel that represents all of the HLA antigens.

If a prospective cardiac transplant recipient's serum tests negative on the lymphocyte panel (a PRA of 0%), we have found that it is unnecessary to perform a crossmatch with a donor before transplantation (a prospective crossmatch). However, in our opinion any patient with detectable anti-HLA antibodies should have a prospective crossmatch to avoid donors with whom a patient might have a hyperacute rejection. Most patients on cardiac transplant recipient lists are stable enough to wait for an appropriate donor rather than taking the first donor available. In lieu of a prospective crossmatch for a patient who has defined antibodies directed against specific HLA antigens, the HLA type of the donor can be obtained and donors with these antigens can be avoided. Occasionally, a patient who has neither been transfused, pregnant, nor previously transplanted will have serum antibodies that react with the lymphocyte panel. In most cases these are autoantibodies that have been induced by the use of procainamide, captopril, hydralazine, or other drugs[15]; these autoantibodies have been found not to have a detrimental effect on transplant outcome. Autoantibodies are predominantly of the immunoglobulin M (IgM) isotype and always react with a patient's own cells as well as with cells from most other individuals.[16] To rule out the concomitant presence of auto- and alloantibodies (the detrimental kind), a patient's serum can be treated with dithiothreitol (DTT), which inactivates IgM but not immunoglobulin G (IgG).[17] Thus, DTT can remove an autoantibody but will leave unaffected alloantibodies, which for practical purposes are of the IgG isotype.

Logistics of the Crossmatch

To perform a crossmatch, the basic ingredients required are the patient's serum, lymphocytes from the donor, and a method of detecting reactivity of the patient's serum with those cells. The most common crossmatching techniques employ a microlymphocytotoxicity technique wherein a small amount of serum is added to donor cells, after which complement and a vital dye are added (see Fig. 2.3).[18] Antibodies that bind complement and react with donor cells will lyse the cells, thus allowing the vital dye to enter. To ensure the detection of antibodies that bind to donor cells but may only weakly bind complement, a more sensitive technique is used in most centers. One such technique employs an antikappa light chain antibody that can bind to human immunoglobulin and activate complement.[19] Thus, noncomplement binding recipient antidonor antibodies can be detected because the antikappa antibody will bind to the recipient's antibodies on the donor's cells and then activate complement, leading to lysis of the cell and entry of the vital dye. These two techniques are known as the standard and antiglobulin crossmatch techniques.

An even more sensitive technique is one using a flow cytometer. A flow cytometer is an instrument that has a laser capable of exciting a fluorochrome attached to an antibody that emits a particle of light that is detectable by a photo multiplier tube. A flow cytometer can analyze each cell as it passes by a window for the presence or absence of a fluorochrome. To exemplify, if a goat antihuman immunoglobulin antibody labeled with either ficoerythrin, which emits a red light upon laser activation, or fluorescein, which emits a green light, is added to donor cells that have previously been incubated with a patient's serum, the cells with recipient antibody attached will be identified upon passage through the flow cytometer. Thus, any amount of patient antibody that is capable of reacting with donor cells will be detected; recipient antibodies capable of causing accelerated graft rejection that might not be detectable using the previously mentioned standard or even antiglobulin techniques may be detectable using the flow cytometer crossmatch technique.[20] There have been cases in which antibodies were not detected using the standard or antiglobulin technique but were detected using a flow cytometer technique and ultimately predicted a poor outcome (unpublished observations of the author). However, because the flow technique is so sensitive it is also capable of identifying antibodies that are not anti-HLA and may not be important to graft outcome. The flow crossmatch does not rely on an antibody's ability to bind complement; however, the flow technique can be used to detect complement binding antibodies. This is accomplished by demonstrating either the release of a fluorochrome from a cell lysed in the presence of complement and antibody or by demonstrating the influx of a fluorochrome into a cell that has been lysed.[21]

Occasionally a patient is in critical condition and in need of the next heart regardless of the result of the crossmatch. However, in most cases this is not true and a prospective crossmatch can be performed. The logistics of performing the prospective crossmatch can be complicated for a donor who is distant from the transplanting center. At the Oregon Health Sciences University we have used a technologist from the Immunogenetics Laboratory who travels with the retrieval team and carries a special kit that includes an inverted stage microscope plus all of the reagents required for a crossmatch (Table 2.1). The crossmatch is then performed on site, using peripheral blood before taking the donor to the operating room. Thus, if the crossmatch is negative for a recipient who has known anti-HLA antibodies, the heart can be taken for that individual. However, if the crossmatch is positive, then the heart can be used for a different recipient who may also have been called into the transplant center. In this way the performance of the crossmatch does not prolong the ischemia time of the donor heart. Moreover, if there is no recipient for which a given center has a crossmatch-negative recipient, then an adjacent transplant center can be alerted to the possibility that a donor heart may be available.

The target cells that are used in the crossmatch are peripheral blood lymphocytes. As previously mentioned, Class I antigens are found on all nucleated cells in the body so lymphocytes will suffice as targets. However, Class II antigens, the DR antigens, are not found on T cells but

TABLE 2.1. Items required for performing a prospective crossmatch away from the transplant center.

1. Inverted phase microscope
2. Centrifuge
3. Recipient serum
4. Reagents
   a. Terasaki ABC trays
   b. Antiglobulin
   c. Thrombin
   d. Lympho-kwik T/B cell
   e. Positive control
   f. Negative control
   g. RPMI
   h. Wash buffer
   i. Eosin
   j. Ficoll hypaque
5. Miscellaneous equipment
   a. Applicator sticks
   b. Aspirating needles
   c. Centrifuge tubes
   d. Cover slips
   e. Fisher tubes
   f. Filters
   g. Forceps
   h. Hamilton syringes
   i. Hemacytometer
   j. Oiled typing trays
   k. Pipettes
   l. Petri dishes
   m. Timer
   n. Test tube rack
   o. Water reservoir
6. Miscellaneous typing worksheets

are found on B cells. Therefore, to detect anti-DR antibodies, a B-cell crossmatch must be performed. In kidney transplantation a positive B-cell crossmatch has been shown to correlate with poorer long-term graft survival[22] and, therefore, many kidney transplant centers include a B-cell crossmatch with the other techniques. In cardiac transplantation no such correlation with a B-cell crossmatch has yet been demonstrated. Therefore, at Oregon Health Sciences University we use only peripheral blood lymphocytes (predominantly T cells) in the crossmatch for heart transplantation. That is, whereas there may be good reason to avoid a donor against whom a recipient has an anti-HLA Class I antibody to date, there is no evidence that it is important to avoid a donor against whom a recipient has an anti-Class II antibody. The tissue distribution of Class II antigens on the transplanted heart is by definition quite limited. The fact that

B cells need not be used in a prospective crossmatch for heart transplantation is fortunate because the techniques for separating B cells from T
cells consumes time and the crossmatching technique using B cells requires longer incubation periods.

Other Aspects of Tissue Typing

Antigen systems other than the HLA system are also important for transplantation. The most important of these is the ABO blood group antigen
system. As is the case with blood transfusions, blood type O donors are
the universal donors and blood type AB individuals are the universal recipients. A blood type A heart cannot be given to a blood type O recipient
but an O heart can be given to an A recipient. There have been cases of
hyperacute rejection occurring when transplantation has been performed
across an incompatible ABO barrier because of naturally occurring antibodies to blood group A and B substances in O individuals.[23] Moreover,
it has become a requirement of the United Network for Organ Sharing
(UNOS, the federally mandated organ procurement and transplantation
network) that O hearts should always go to O recipients, A to A, and B
to B. It is felt that this will prevent the under utilization of A and B hearts
that could go unused if O hearts are given to A and B recipients indiscrim-
inately. This would lead to a build-up of blood type O recipients on waiting lists. Matching for Lewis[24] antigens in kidney transplantation may be
of some benefit but this is not practical in heart or liver transplantation.

Basic Immunology

The immune system consists of both nonspecific and specific components
(see Table 2.2). The nonspecific system consists of cells that are involved
with (1) phagocytosis, (2) presentation of antigens to cells involved with
specific immunity, and (3) mediation of inflammation by release of a variety of cytoplasmic products that mediate inflammation. The cellular components of the nonspecific immunity system are polymorphonuclear cells,
basophils, eosinophils, monocytes, tissue macrophages, some vascular
endothelial cells, and platelets. These cells are involved with protecting
the body's various portals of entry from invasion by microorganisms.
Whereas all of these components can be important in mediating organ
allograft rejection, it has been demonstrated that immunosuppression directed specifically to T cells appears to be sufficient for blocking an allograft response.[25,26] Nevertheless, if the cells of the specific immune response are not blocked, then the allograft rejection response can recruit
all of the abovementioned components into an allograft.

Specific immunity is mediated by lymphocytes, T cells, and B cells (see
Fig. 2.5). T cells are the primary initiators of the immune response; T

TABLE 2.2. Effectors of the immune system.

Nonspecific effectors	Specific effectors
Antigen-presenting cells	Humoral immunity
Macrophages	Complement-dependent antibody-mediated
Dendritic cells	cytotoxicity
Endothelial cells	Immune complex formation
Phagocytic cells	Opsonization
Monocytes/macrophates	Cell-mediated immunity
Polymorphonuclear cells	T-cell cytotoxicity
Eosinophils	Delayed-type hypersensitivity
Cytokines	Natural killer cells
Interleukins	
Histamine	
SRS-A	

helper cells are activated first by antigens-presented to them by the accessory cells of the immune response. As previously mentioned, accessory cells, or antigen-presenting cells, are monocytes, tissue macrophages, and in some cases vascular endothelial cells. The activation of a helper cell requires both antigen and soluble signal from the antigen-presenting cell, an interleukin called IL-1. T helper cells generally cannot be activated unless an antigen is presented in the context of its own HLA Class II antigens. The importance of accessory cells can be demonstrated in vitro in a mixed lymphocyte culture; pure donor T cells cannot be activated by pure donor B cells without macrophages. Either donor or recipient macrophages can provide the ingredients necessary to activate T cells. This suggests that in organ transplantation, donor passenger macrophages and dendritic cells may be capable of directly stimulating recipient helper T cells. Thus, passenger leukocytes may be capable of providing both of the necessary signals for T cell activation, antigen, and a soluble interleukin; donor Class II antigens are probably mistakenly recognized as self Class II plus antigen. This may also be true for donor Class I antigens. Donor leukocytes that are incapable of providing the second, soluble signal probably are not important initiators of the immune response except by providing Class I and Class II antigens to be processed by host antigen presenting cells.

Activation of a T helper cell results in expression of interleukin-2 receptors and production of interleukin-2, a soluble factor also known as T-cell growth factor (TCGF); interleukin-2 is required for further activation of T cells. By releasing interleukin-2, T helper cells activate clones of cytotoxic T cells that are capable of reacting specifically with foreign polypeptides on Class I and Class II antigens, as well as against minor histocompatibility antigens. T helper cells are also able to activate B cells by releasing other interleukins that stimulate B-cell growth and differentia-

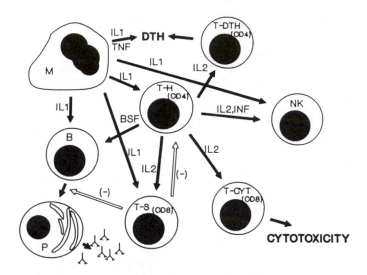

FIGURE 2.5. Specific effectors of the immunologic response. The macrophage (M) presents antigen to the T helper cell (T-H) along with IL-1, which results in stimulation and clonal expansion. The T helper can differentiate into T cells involved in delayed-type hypersensitivity reactions (T-DTH) as well as stimulate the recruitment of natural killer cells (NK), T suppressor cells (T-S), and cytotoxic cells (T-CYT). In addition, the T helper cell, via the release of a variety of cytokines including IL-4 (BSF, B-cell stimulation factor), results in the expansion and differentiation of B lymphocytes (B) into plasma cells (P), resulting in the production of antibody.

tion, and can further activate certain T cells and null cells, or "killer cells", by releasing gamma interferon.

The basic mechanisms of immunity that are mediated by the specific immune response are cellular- and antibody-based. Three forms of cell-based immunity can occur: (1) T-cell cytotoxicity, wherein the T cell deals a lethal hit to a target cell to which it has attached, causing essentially no damage to surrounding tissues; (2) delayed-type hypersensitivity, wherein tissue damage is mediated by T-cell and macrophage release of toxic products, and (3) natural killer cells that are thought to participate in a more nonspecific fashion in tumor cell surveillance and can also react against virally infected cells. This reaction is not directed to a specific viral polypeptide sequence but rather to glycoprotein components that all viruses have in common. Antibody-mediated immunity is almost always specifically directed to foreign antigen. However, there can also be autoantibody-mediated processes such as those found in systemic lupus erythematosus. Antibody-mediated immunity relies on the ability of antibody to activate complement or by aggregated immunoglobulin to activate directly other cells that are capable of mediating an inflammatory reaction.

A final form of immunity uses both antibodies and cells and is known as antibody-dependent cell-mediated cytotoxicity; certain cells called null cells or killer cells can bind to the Fc portion of an immunoglobulin molecule that has bound to a target cell. The subsequent release of toxic products by these cells results in the death of the target cell. The importance of this mechanism in mediating allograft rejection is not well known.

T cells and B cells are capable of reacting against only one specific polypeptide sequence (antigen) perceived as nonself. Therefore, during any given immune response only a small number of cells undergo clonal expansion and react to the target antigen or antigens. In the case of an allograft response, there may be several different donor polypeptides that are recognized as nonself; several cells may undergo clonal expansion as a result. Many cells may be nonspecifically recruited by interleukin-2 and other cytokines to proliferate, but only those programmed to react with the foreign antigen on the target molecules will be capable of mediating the immune response.

The T-cell receptor for antigen is the equivalent of an antibody; it is programmed to react with a single target. T-cell receptors of any single cell and its cloned offspring are identical. The amazing thing about the specific immune response is that there are antibodies and T cell receptors capable of reacting with so many different antigens. The potential nonself antigens number in the millions; there are simply not enough genes in the human genome to code for all of the different antibodies and T-cell receptors that would be required to recognize each unique antigen. Instead, an incredible antibody and T-cell receptor diversity is possible because of the presence of multiple genes capable of rearranging and combining in millions of different ways, leading to the millions of different unique peptides in the hypervariable regions on antibodies and T-cell receptors. To our knowledge, the gene regions coding for these structures are the only ones capable of this sort of rearrangement.

Immunopathogenesis of Rejection

Rejection of a transplanted organ can be mediated by both antibodies and cells. In general, antibody-mediated rejection is the more serious because once antibodies are present in an allograft there is little that can be done to reverse the inflammatory process that they initiate. On the other hand, the immunosuppression armamentarium possessed by most transplant centers contains drugs that are fully capable of reversing cell-mediated rejections. The most devastating form of antibody-mediated rejection is that mediated by antidonor antibodies that are present in the patient's serum at the time of transplantation. This form of rejection is known as hyperacute rejection and can lead to immediate graft failure. If present in sufficient quantities, antidonor antibodies combine with Class I antigens present in abundant amounts on vascular endothelium in the heart. An irreversible sequence of events ensues, consisting of complement activation, platelet adherence and aggregation, fibrin deposition, vessel occlusion, myocardial ischemia, and eventual necrosis and fatal arrythmia or heart failure. A more subacute form of initial antibody-mediated rejection is one that results in an arteritis, which can have the same outcome but in a more protracted fashion.

Hyperacute rejection is rare in cardiac transplantation because it is unusual for a potential heart transplant patient to have received the necessary stimuli to develop anti-HLA antibodies. However, patients with prior open heart surgery may have received blood transfusions, some women may have had multiple pregnancies, or some patients may have had a prior heart transplantation. All of these can stimulate anti-HLA antibody production and if anti-HLA antibodies are present, the only way to avoid hyperacute rejection is to perform a prospective crossmatch. Under certain circumstances it may also be possible to remove these antidonor antibodies by employing a technique of plasmapheresis or by passing patient serum over a column that specifically removes immunoglobulin. These latter techniques are investigational at present. In contrast to the situation in heart transplantation, in kidney transplantation hyperacute rejections could occur frequently because patients with renal failure are often anemic and require multiple blood transfusions. Therefore, the crossmatch is extremely important in the setting of kidney transplantation.

Antibodies that develop after transplantation may be involved with another more insidious type of rejection known as chronic rejection.[27] In cardiac transplantation, chronic rejection is manifest by accelerated atherosclerosis that develops as a result of antibody- (and possibly cellular) mediated damage of coronary artery endothelium; this reduces natural defenses against cholesterol deposition and platelet adherence and promotes vascular smooth muscle cell proliferation.

Cell-mediated rejection is the most common form of rejection encountered immediately after transplantation; most patients develop one or more episodes of this after transplantation. These rejection episodes tend to come in waves during the first six months after transplantation and in general are successfully treated with antirejection immunotherapy. The basic cellular mechanisms involved with acute rejection episodes include direct T-cell cytotoxicity and delayed-type hypersensitivity mediated by T cells and macrophages. Natural killer cells might also be involved with the rejection response but their role is less well defined. During an acute rejection episode, both cytotoxic and helper T cells can be found in an allograft.[28] In the peripheral blood the ratio of helper to cytotoxic cells is generally approximately 2 : 1; in a rejection allograft that ratio is often reversed owing to the predominance of cytotoxic cells mediating rejection reactions. There have been many experimental studies using nonhuman transplant models that have attempted to establish the relative importance of delayed-type hypersensitivity reactions (CD4 initiated) and direct T-cell cytotoxicity (CD8 mediated) in acute rejection of allografts. These studies have not been conclusive but they do indicate that cells of the helper or CD4 phenotype appear to be of equal importance to cells of the cytotoxic or CD8 phenotype.[29]

Conclusions

Advancing our knowledge of the immune response as it relates to transplantation will probably result in major innovations in immunotherapy for transplantation in the next decade. If improved cardiac preservation techniques can be developed, transplant programs may also be able to capitalize on the advantages that would accompany better HLA antigen matching.

References

1. Hood L, Weissman I, Wood W, Wilson J. Genes and proteins of the major histocompatibility complex. In: Hood L, Weissman I, Wood W, Wilson J, eds. *Immunology*. Menlo Park, Calif: The Benjamin/Cummings Publishing Co Inc; 1984:189–190.
2. Thomas AJ, Hildreth JEK. Proteins and the molecular basis of cell mediated immunity. In: Williams G, Melvill H, Burdick J, Solez K, eds. *Kidney Transplant Rejection, Diagnosis and Treatment*. New York, NY: Marcel Dekker Inc; 1986:3–5.
3. Cho YW, Terasa P. Long-term survival. In: Terasaki P, ed. *Clinical Transplant 1988*. Los Angeles, The Regents of the University of California; 1988:277–282.
4. DeWolf W, O'Leary J, Yunis E. Cellular typing. In: Rose N, Friedman H, eds. *Manual of Clinical Immunology*. Washington, DC: Am Soc Microbiol; 1980:1007–1028
5. Banner N, Fitzgerald M, Khaghani D, et al. Cardiac transplantation at Harefield Hospital. In: Terasaki P, ed. *Clinical Transplants 1987*. Los Angeles, The Regents of University of California; 1987:24–26.
6. Nossal GJV. Current concepts: immunology of the basic components of the immune system. *N Engl J Med*. 1987;316:1320–1325
7. Hood L, Weissman I, Wood W, Wilson J. The immune response. In: Hood L, Weissman I, Wood W, Wilson J, eds. *Immunology*. Menlo Park, Calif: The Benjamin/Cummings Publishing Co Inc; 1984:296–297.
8. Dupont B. Nomenclature for factors of the HLA system, 1987. *Hum Immunol*. 1989;26:3–14.

9. Dausset J, Cohen D. HLA at the gene level. In: Albert ED, Baur MP, Mayr WR, eds. *Histocompatibility Testing 1984*. Heidelberg: Springer-Verlag; 1984:22–27.

10. Bidwell J. DNA-RFLP analysis and genotyping of HLA-DR and DQ antigens. *Immunol Today*. 1988;9:18–22.

11. DeWolf W, O'Leary J, Yunis E. Cellular typing. In: Rose N, Friedman H, eds. *Manual of Clinical Immunology*. Washington, DC: Am Soc Microbiol; 1980:1018–1022.

12. Hood L, Weissman I, Wood W, Wilson J. Tissue transplantation. In: Hood L, Weissman I, Wood W, Wilson J, eds. *Immunology*. Menlo Park, Calif: The Benjamin/Cummings Publishing Inc; 1984:403–408.

13. Kissmeyer-Nielson F, Olsens, Peterson VP, Fjeldborg O. Hyperacute rejection of kidney allograft, associated with pre-existing humoral antibodies against donor cells. *Lancet*. 1988;2:662–665.

14. Marshall WH, Barnard JM. Joint report, A2. In: Terasaki P, ed. *Histocompatibility Testing 1980*. Los Angeles, The Regents of the University of California; 1980:293–295.

15. McNamara C, Braun WE, Zachary AA, et al. Autolymphocytotoxins in cardiac transplantation: serology, significance and association with HLA-A1 and HLA-A3. In: Dupont BO, ed. *Immunology of HLA. Immunogenetics and Histocompatibility*. New York, NY: Springer-Verlag; 1989;II:532–533.

16. Lobo P. Nature of autolymphocytotoxins present in renal hemodialysis patients. *Transplantation*. 1981;32:233–237.

17. Chapman JE, Taylor CJ, Ting A, Morris PJ. Immunoglobulin class and specificity of antibodies causing positive T cell crossmatches. Relationship to renal transplant outcome. *Transplantation*. 1986;42:608–613.

18. NIAID, Staff Report. NIH lymphocyte microcytotoxicity technique. In: *NIAID, Manual of Tissue Typing Techniques 1976–1977*. Washington, D.C., Department of Health, Education, and Welfare; 1976:22–24.

19. Fuller TC, Cosimi AB, Russel PS. Use of an antiglobulin-ATG reagent for detection of low levels of alloantibody-improvements of allograft survival in presensitized recipients. *Transplant Proc*. 1978;10:436–465.

20. Garovoy MR, Rheinschmidt MA, Bigos M, et al. Flow cytometry analysis: a high technology crossmatch technique facilitating transplantation. *Transplant Proc*. 1983;XV:1939–1944.

21. Wetzsteon PJ, Head MA, Fletcher LA, Norman DJ. Cytotoxic flow crossmatches. *Hum Immunol* September 1989;44. Abstract.

22. Noreen H, van der Hagen E, Segall M, et al. Renal allograft survival in patient with positive donor specific B lymphocyte crossmatches. *Transplant Proc*. 1983;15:1216–1217.

23. Wilbrandt R, Tung K. ABO blood group incompatibility in human renal homotransplantation. *Am J Clin Pathol*. 1969;15:15–23.

24. Roy R, Terasaki PI, Chia D, Mickey M. Low kidney graft survival in Lewis negative patients after regrafting and newer matching schemes for Lewis. *Transplant Proc*. 1987;19:4498–4502.

25. Millis M, Busutill R. Ramdomized prospective trial of OKT*3 for early prophylaxis of rejection after liver transplantation. *Transplantation*. 1989;47: 82–88.

26. Ortho Multicenter Transplant Study Group. A randomized clinical trial of

OKT*3 monoclonal antibody for acute rejection of cadaveric renal transplants. *N Engl J Med*. 1985;313:337–342.
27. Cabrol C, Aupetit B. Current problems in cardiac transplantation. In: Terasaki P, ed. *Clinical Transplants 1987*. Los Angeles, The Regents of the University of California; 1987:27–31.
28. Yacoub MH, Gracie JA, Rose ML, Cox J, Fraser AK, Chisholm PM. T cell characterization in human cardiac allografts. *Transplantation*. 1983;38:634–637.
29. Hall B, deSaxe I, Dorsch S. The cellular basis of allograft rejection in vivo. *Transplantation*. 1983;36:700–705.

3
Medical Therapy Tailored for Advanced Heart Failure

LYNNE WARNER STEVENSON

The success of transplantation has encouraged referrals to transplant centers, where the supply of donor hearts is so limited that most patients cannot undergo transplantation, and those who are accepted frequently have long waiting periods.[1,2] The concentration of uniquely compromised patients at these centers has led to the development of therapy specifically tailored for advanced heart failure. This chapter will discuss the physiology of advanced heart failure and the principles of acute and chronic therapy to improve status both in patients awaiting transplantation and in the many patients who are ineligible for transplantation.

The Presentation and Physiology of Heart Failure

More than 90% of patients referred for transplantation have dilated ventricular failure that has evolved over months or years in most cases but occasionally presents with rapid decompensation from massive infarction, acute myocarditis, or open-heart surgery. The restrictive cardiomyopathies and other uncommon etiologies of heart failure without severe left ventricular systolic dysfunction will not be directly addressed in this chapter.

Many patients with low ejection fractions are well compensated hemodynamically and functionally, and are able to continue with regular employment and activities. Their original myocardial injury has led to ventricular hypertrophy and dilatation such that resting hemodynamics are within normal limits, while the decrease in maximal function is unappreciated due to unrecognized activity restriction. The prevalence and persistence of effective compensation with low ejection fraction is probably underestimated. Such patients occasionally may come to attention after symptomatic arrhythmias, embolic events, or incidental chest x-rays showing cardiomegaly. Careful evaluation should be performed to identify potentially reversible insults, such as silent ischemia and excessive alcohol consumption, and risk factors for early death, such as sustained ventricular arrhythmias and critical coronary disease. If such patients have at least Class II exercise capacity documented by oxygen consumption and anaerobic threshold measurement, and do not have high risk factors for early mortality, we do not evaluate further for transplantation but maintain close supervision. Current evidence suggests that vasodilator therapy may prolong survival in this population, perhaps by preventing further ventricular dilatation and the development of secondary mitral regurgitation, which is important also after large myocardial infarction.[3,4]

Many patients whose ventricular dysfunction after major infarction, myocarditis, or toxic insult is initially compensated exhibit later deterioration even without continued primary injury. Alterations at the level of the individual myocyte, in integrated cardiac function, and in systemic circulatory adaptation all contribute to progressive decompensation.

At the cellular level, there are decreased numbers and response of beta-adrenergic receptors and guanine nucleotide-binding regulatory proteins.[5,6] It is not known yet whether the altered proportions of oxidative and glycolytic enzymes[7] are adaptive or detrimental. Calcium uptake and release is affected[8] and adenosine triphosphate (ATP) metabolism may be reduced or abnormally compartmentalized.[9]

Global cardiac function is altered in multiple ways. The primary decrease in systolic function is accompanied by an increase in ventricular volume. Whereas the resulting ventricular hypertrophy initially may be adequate to maintain normal wall stress, further dilatation cannot be accommodated and the wall stress increases markedly, first owing to the factor of the increased radius and later in the course of disease owing also to the increasing filling pressures. Ventricular dilatation may in some cases even be disproportionate to the volume overload if the connective tissue architecture has been disrupted by the primary injury.

Marked ventricular dilatation leads to mitral regurgitation, which is related to the ventricular size and in some cases also to secondary mitral annular and left atrial dilatation. In patients with coronary artery disease, ischemia or infarction of papillary muscles and the supporting ventricular wall contribute to mitral regurgitation. Regardless of the etiology of dilated heart failure, mitral regurgitation diverts a significant proportion of total ventricular stroke volume by the time severe symptoms of congestion have developed, as demonstrated in patients referred for transplantation.[10] Mitral regurgitation then contributes further to the volume overload of the left ventricle. Although the elevated afterload faced by the failing left ventricle is frequently equated with the systemic arterial resistance (see below), it should be recognized that, before beginning ejection, the ventricle must also overcome the load posed by the end-diastolic volume and pressure, which could be considered the internal afterload.[11]

Severe left heart failure is frequently accompanied by right heart failure. Whereas right ventricular involvement at the time of initial diagnosis may be more common in patients with primary cardiomyopathy, patients with chronic left ventricular failure presenting for cardiac transplantation commonly have severe right heart failure regardless of initial etiology. Secondary development of right heart failure presumably occurs as a result of chronically elevated pulmonary pressures, similar to that with longstanding mitral stenosis. Patients with more reactive pulmonary hypertension may develop right heart failure sooner. Right ventricular dilatation leads to tricuspid regurgitation, which also becomes a major drain from forward cardiac output. In addition, the transmission of elevated right-sided pressures into the systemic venous circulation may be more important than the depressed forward output in the development of malnutrition and "cardiac cachexia".[12]

Systemic responses to altered cardiac function in the advanced stages of disease initially may preserve and subsequently impair overall cardiovascular function. Fluid retention in excess of that required for optimal cardiac filling results in part from the blunted inhibition of renal sympathetic tone after chronic atrial dilatation.[13] Detrimental fluid retention often precedes clinical evidence of inadequate perfusion and contributes to the ventricular dilatation and congestive symptoms. Activation of sympathetic reflexes from decreased perfusion causes increased large artery impedance and peripheral vascular resistance, which increases the ventricular afterload.[14] The renin-angiotensin system is active systemically to cause vasoconstriction and fluid retention, and is also localized within regional vascular beds.[15] Vasopressin levels are elevated in some patients, increasing vascular resistance and thirst while decreasing water excretion and modulating other reflex responses.[16] Atrial natriuretic factor secretion, increased in response to atrial and ventricular stretch, is not in itself adequate to counteract opposing sympathetic activity but may contribute to the balance between fluid retention and excretion.[17] The physiologic importance of other circulating hormones such as vasointestinal peptide and endothelin have not yet been established.

Prognosis at the Time of Referral

The varying degrees of cardiac, circulatory, and neurohumoral derangements evident in the individual patient referred with heart failure for transplantation will influence prognosis and therapy. Although most referring physicians consider their patients to be end-stage, it is valuable to attempt to discriminate more carefully at the time of initial evaluation. By the time dilated heart failure is advanced and ejection fraction is less than 0.25, the ejection fraction itself is of less value in prognosis than when more diverse populations are followed. The limited usefulness of the ejection fraction in this range may reflect the limitations of measurement, the inclusion of regurgitant ejection in the total ejection fraction, and the relatively increasing importance of other adaptive and maladaptive responses. Ventricular size independent of etiology has not been shown to be of major prognostic

TABLE 3.1. Profile of 150 patients with ejection fraction ≤20% at time of referral for transplantation.

Age (years)	45 ± 13
Clinical class (NYHA)[a]	3.6 ± 0.5
Hospitalizations (no. previous 6 mos)	2 ± 2
Left ventricular ejection fraction	15 ± 3%
Left ventricular diameter (diastolic, mm)	76 ± 10
Cardiac index (L/min/m²)	2.0 ± 0.6
Pulmonary wedge pressure (mmHg)	28 ± 9
Pulmonary arterial systolic pressure (mmHg)	55 ± 16
Right atrial pressure (mmHg)	13 ± 9
Mean arterial pressure (mmHg)	84 ± 10
Systemic vascular resistance (dynes-sec-cm⁻⁵)	1700 ± 700

[a]NYHA = New York Heart Association.

value, although this may be due in part to the frequent combination of ischemic heart failure patients with nonischemic cardiomyopathy patients, who tend to have bigger ventricles and better prognosis. Clinical class has not useful in the population referred for transplant, most of whom demonstrate greater than Class III limitation and low maximum oxygen consumption on exercise testing, which can often be modified after more aggressive medical therapy. The typical population with low ejection fraction referred for transplantation is outlined in Table 3.1.

Serum norepinephrine levels have been helpful in broad populations,[18] but are almost always elevated in the advanced heart failure population, in whom the degree of elevation has been less helpful. Serum sodium and renin levels have been helpful even in populations restricted to severe disease, reflecting the importance of neurohumoral activity.[19] Low triiodothyronine and elevated reverse triiodothyronine and their ratio have been found to be very potent predictors of mortality in the severely ill heart failure population, which may merely reflect a combination of negative factors or themselves contribute to worsening cardiac and systemic function.[20]

Hemodynamic parameters, such as cardiac index, and pulmonary capillary wedge pressure have been described as predictors of mortality in heart failure.[21,22] However, they are almost always abnormal in the patients referred for transplantation (Table 3.1). The degree of hemodynamic derangement appears to reflect the inadequacy of previous treatment in addition to the severity of underlying disease, which can be better determined after therapy specifically tailored to approach normal hemodynamics in this population.

Afterload Reduction Tailored for Hemodynamic Goals

The referral for transplantation of patients with low ejection fraction and severe symptoms of heart failure is frequently considered a defeat for medical therapy. However, many such patients are not truly "refrac-

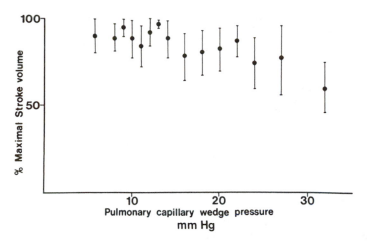

FIGURE 3.1. Maintenance of maximal stroke volume with normal filling pressures in 20 patients with advanced heart failure (ejection fraction <25%) during tailored therapy with intravenous nitroprusside and diuretics.

tory,'' despite previous therapy with digitalis, diuretics, and vasodilators as generally used in the community. These patients can still derive major benefit from medical therapy specifically tailored to advanced heart failure.[23] Previous therapy reflected assumptions derived from populations with acute failure or chronic milder left ventricular dysfunction. In contrast, patients with severe congestive symptoms from chronic dilated ventricular failure have recently been attracted and concentrated in transplant centers, allowing elucidation of the unique principles that apply to this population. The new approach includes the realization that the immediate goals are not merely improved hemodynamics, but normal hemodynamics, with particular attention to filling pressures. Such goals can be established only by therapy that is tailored individually to hemodynamic measurements for each patient because hemodynamic status and drug responses cannot be predicted reliably from routine physical examination.[24]

Aggressive therapy to lower ventricular filling pressures with vasodilators and diuretics in heart failure has been restricted by concern that cardiac output will be compromised further if high filling pressures are not maintained. The chronically dilated left ventricle, however, differs from the acutely ischemic ventricle or stiff restricted ventricle. Sarcomere length is already maximal, with further ventricular dilation allowed by defective connective tissue structure and slippage. Maximal cardiac outputs in chronically dilated ventricles are frequently achieved at normal filling pressures, even in patients with previous marked elevations in filling pressures,[25] as shown in Figure 3.1. The improvement in cardiac output that accompanies reduction of ventricular filling pressures and volumes results largely from the decrease in mitral regurgitation,[26] which is

TABLE 3.2. Tailored therapy for advanced heart failure.

1. Measurement of baseline hemodynamics
2. Intravenous nitroprusside and diuretics tailored to hemodynamic goals:
   PCW[a]≤15 mmHg
   SVR[b]≤1200 dynes-sec-cm^{-5}
   RA[c]≤8 mmHg
   SBP[d]≥80 mmHg
3. Definition of optimal hemodynamics by 24–48 hr
4. Titration of high-dose oral vasodilators as nitroprusside weaned:
   Maximum doses: Captopril 400 mg/day
   Hydralazine 400 mg/day
   Isosorbide 320 mg/day
5. Ambulation, diuretic adjustment for 24–48 hr
6. Maintain digoxin if no contraindication
7. Detailed patient education
8. Flexible outpatient diuretic regimen
9. Progressive walking program
10. Vigilant follow-up

[a]PCW = pulmonary capillary wedge pressure.
[b]SVR = systemic vascular resistance.
[c]RA = right atrial pressure.
[d]SBP = systolic blood pressure.

significant in almost all patients with severe heart failure, regardless of whether the characteristic murmur is detected.[10]

Systemic vascular resistance has frequently been targeted in reduction of the afterload faced by the failing ventricle. However, this is only the external afterload. The ventricle must also face the internal afterload[11] increased by ventricular dilatation and further increased by mitral regurgitation. The distinction between preload and afterload reduction is thus blurred, as the ventricular afterload includes the preload. The use of diuretics and vasodilators to reduce ventricular filling pressures is actually a major aspect of true afterload reduction, as well as preload reduction. Congestive symptoms are not only unnecessary in most patients with heart failure, but they usually indicate elevated filling pressures, which add to myocardial energy demands and may hasten ventricular decompensation. In addition, elevated right ventricular pressures and tricuspid regurgitation contribute to malnutrition, which further compromises cardiac and systemic status.[12]

Therapy for patients referred with advanced heart failure as outlined in Table 3.2 is tailored to the hemodynamic goals of near-normal filling pressures while maintaining systolic blood pressures greater than 80 mmHg,[23,26] which is usually well tolerated by the typical transplant candidate (≤65 years old). Intravenous agents are used first, usually nitroprusside and occasionally intravenous nitroglycerin, simultaneously with intravenous loop diuretics (furosemide, bumetanide, or rarely ethacrynic acid). Addition of oral thiazides, the most potent of which is metolazone, potentiates the effect of loop diuretics because of their action on the distal tubule as well as possibly potentiating their proximal tubular effects.[27] After hemodynamic goals have been achieved on intravenous agents, oral vasodilators and diuretics are added as nitroprusside is tapered. High doses of oral vasodilators are often required to maintain the hemodynamics achieved. Either captopril or hydralazine are used initially with occasional substitution with enalapril in very stable patients. Hydralazine is the agent most likely to achieve the hemodynamic goals without causing severe hypotension in the sickest patients, although side effects (nausea) occasionally may limit its use. Patients are then discharged on oral vasodilators, digoxin to maintain levels of 1.0 to 2.0 ng/ml unless contraindicated, and oral loop diuretics with additional metolazone to be taken for weight gain that does not resolve after doubling the furosemide dose.

Tailored therapy has allowed hospital discharge in 80% of patients referred for urgent transplantation.[23] We have since employed this therapy in all patients referred with severe symptoms; for the last ˙150 patients referred with ejection fractions ≤20% and initial status as shown in Table 3.1, tailored therapy allowed 63% 1-year survival without transplantation. In contrast to previous data, the hemodynamic parameters *at the time of referral* did not predict survival in this population. The major hemodynamic risk factor for death after tailored therapy was a pulmonary capillary wedge pressure that could not be reduced to less than 16 mmHg. (The presence of severe coronary artery disease was an additional risk factor for early death, regardless of hemodynamic status.)

Tailored afterload reduction initially establishes adequate perfusion and freedom from congestive symptoms in approximately 90% of patients referred to transplantation by cardiologists from a typical major metropolitan and surrounding rural area (Fig. 3.2). Initial failure of tailored therapy cannot be predicted reliably for an individual patient by any of these parameters at the time of referral, although it is more common in those patients with worse initial sodium, renal, and hepatic function.[23]

Most adults in whom hemodynamic stability cannot be established even for a short time without nonglycosidic inotropic therapy or mechanical support are patients who have had a recent acute insult such as a myocardial infarction, cardiopulmonary bypass, or acute myocarditis (defined by duration <6 weeks rather than by histological criteria). Patients with acute decompensation caused by inappropriate therapy with negative inotropic drugs may require combination intravenous inotropic therapy temporarily but can generally be rescued without resorting to mechanical assistance. Experience with pediatric patients is limited, but we have found patients who are younger than 20 years old to be much more likely to develop refractory decompensation without apparent precipitating cause after chronic stable heart failure, which appears to be associated with disproportionate right ventricular compromise in this group.

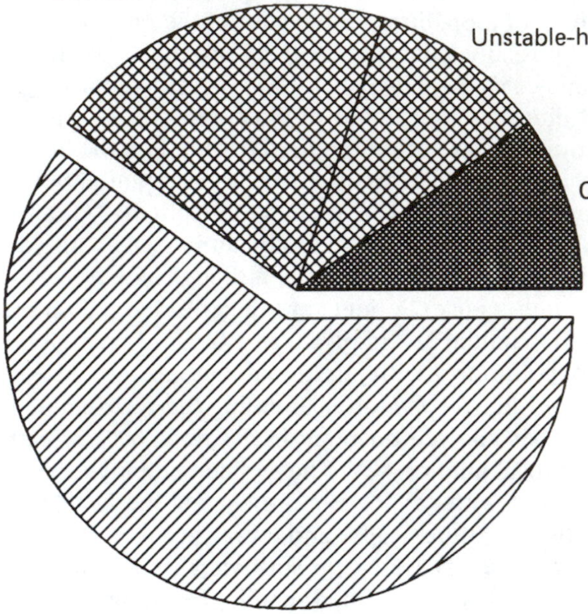

Unstable-home 20%

Unstable-hospital 10%

Critical 10%

Stable 60%

FIGURE 3.2. Clinical status after tailored medical therapy in patients with advanced heart failure referred for cardiac transplantation.

The Stepped Approach to Therapy for Critical Patients

For adult and pediatric patients who are refractory to tailored afterload reduction with aggressive vasodilators and diuretics, subsequent therapy should be instituted in progressively escalating steps (Fig.3.3). Intravenous inotropic therapy facilitates the diuresis necessary to reverse the cycle of increasing ventricular volumes and regurgitation, and frequently may be tapered after several days, allowing subsequent maintenance on oral vasodilators and diuretics alone. Tapering is most likely to be possible when partial agonists such as dobutamine and dopamine in low doses have been employed. Low doses of these and all inotropic agents should be used initially to minimize resulting modifications in the adrenergic receptor-guanine nucleotide binding protein-adenylate cyclase complex,[28] which may increase dependence on exogenous inotropic agents.

In addition to stimulation of heart rate and contractility, dobutamine and dopamine are both vasodilators at doses ≤3 μg/kg, due to beta$_2$ stimulation, and for dopamine, stimulation of dopamine receptors. Dobutamine remains a vasodilator at all doses, but at higher doses dopamine causes vasoconstriction due to dominant alpha-receptor stimulation and release

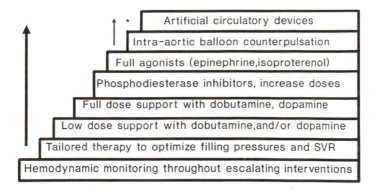

FIGURE 3.3. The Stepped Approach to stabilization of patients with critically compromised hemodynamic status before cardiac transplantation. *Patients without ischemia may be considered for circulatory assist devices other than the intraaortic balloon pump after failure of pharmacologic steps. SVR = systemic vascular resistance.

of endogenous norepinephrine stores. Unlike dobutamine, dopamine activates dopamine receptors, which cause renal vasodilatation without overriding alpha stimulation, so the addition of "renal-dose" dopamine (<5 μg/kg/min) to dobutamine may in some cases aid diuresis.

In general, rapid escalation to higher steps of therapy is indicated when hypoperfusion causes increasing lactate production or mental obtundation, or when pulmonary congestion compromises adequate ventilation despite high oxygen concentrations and preload reduction with intravenous nitrates and diuretics (and potentially dialysis). As renal and hepatic failure will not generally reverse rapidly, they are indications for escalation of therapy over hours rather than minutes.

The newer inotropic agents such as intravenous amrinone and milrinone appear to act primarily by inhibiting phosphodiesterase, thus initially bypassing the beta receptor complex, which is down-regulated by standard nonglycosidic inotropic agents. They thus frequently increase inotropy further when added to these other inotropic agents. There is concern that this increased inotropy may be paid for by subsequent further myocardial depression through unknown mechanisms.[29] Increased cyclic AMP also causes vasodilation, which in some patients may be the predominant effect of phosphodiesterase inhibitors and may necessitate some decrease in concomitant vasodilators. Compensatory decrease in response results after use of the phosphodiesterase inhibitors, perhaps as a result of decreased adrenergic response to intrinsic catecholamines.[30]

Judicious use of intravenous phosphodiesterase inhibitors frequently allows hospital stabilization of patients who might otherwise receive mechanical assist devices. This pharmacologic "bridging" to transplant (specifically described for enoximone, by Loisance) avoids the infectious and hematologic risks associated with in-dwelling prosthetic materials and in some cases thoracotomy. Although doses of as high as 15 to 20 μg/kg per min have been used, the lowest dose necessary should be employed, after a loading dose of 0.75mg/kg. Minimizing the dose reduces the risk of thrombocytopenia and liver dysfunction, which occur frequently with intravenous amrinone, currently the only widely available agent of this type. In addition, the use of the lowest possible dose minimizes the intracellular adaptations that compromise subsequent weaning, and also leaves a larger margin for later increases that may be necessary. Titration and weaning of phosphodiesterase inhibitors is much more difficult than for other intravenous inotropic agents because of their potency and prolonged half-life. Many patients who initially appear to tolerate weaning will demonstrate rapid and sometimes irreversible decompensation 16 to 48 hours later. Although these agents can be extremely valuable, the difficulties and dangers in their use and weaning have led us to reserve them only for patients who have failed adequate trial of the previous steps, as has been advised.[29] It has been our experience that patients who truly required phosphodiesterase inhibitors can seldom be subsequently weaned, remaining on intravenous phosphodiesterase inhibitor support until transplantation, death, or the institution of other experimental therapy.

Institution of the full adrenergic agonist isoproterenol, which stimulates heart rate, contractility, and peripheral vasodilation through beta receptors, or epinephrine, which stimulates heart rate and contractility with a net vasoconstriction due to stimulation of both alpha and beta receptors, is usually reserved for patients who have not responded adequately to phosphodiesterase inhibitors, although it may occasionally be tried earlier. Although these potent agents can markedly increase arrhythmias and myocardial ischemia, they should be tried before insertion of total artificial support. Norepinephrine increases heart rate and contractility but also causes more vasoconstriction than epinephrine and is generally reserved for patients with excessive vasodilation, such as those with concomitant sepsis or chronic liver failure.

Patients should always be evaluated for myocardial ischemia early in the course of circulatory decompensation. Whereas the role of microcirculatory compromise in patients without large vessel coronary artery disease is unclear, patients with presumed ischemia from discrete stenoses, or from inadequate collateralization of areas distal to complete coronary occlusions, should be considered for immediate placement of an intraaortic balloon before prolonged pharmacologic trials. It should be emphasized that the placement of such a device should be considered an interim procedure because it seldom improves outcome without subsequent definitive therapy such as transplantation, emergency angioplasty, or in some cases coronary artery bypass surgery despite poor ejection fraction.[31,32]

Inflation of the balloon in the descending aorta during diastole augments coronary perfusion, and deflation during systole decreases ventricular afterload and cardiac work. The major benefit appears to derive from the effects on coronary perfusion, which may make support with inotropic agents or total artificial devices unnecessary if compromise has been related to ischemia. Such patients often require continued support until transplantation can be performed, although weaning should periodically be attempted. The benefit of balloon counterpulsation without obvious ischemia is less clear. Rapid weaning and removal has been possible without apparent deterioration in most patients with nonischemic cardiomyopathy who have been transferred on intraaortic balloon pumps. The risk of systemic infection and limb ischemia during prolonged central instrumentation is high and must be weighed against the evidence of hemodynamic benefit. The systemic anticoagulation that most consider important to avoid thrombosis is associated with its own risk of hemorrhage. Less common complications are thrombocytopenia, aortic dissection, and balloon malfunction. The intraaortic balloon should not be placed in patients with aortic insufficiency or dissecting aneurysm.

The intraaortic balloon is inserted over a guidewire through a sheath in a peripheral large artery (unless inserted directly during cardiac surgery), usually the femoral artery, into the descending aorta distal to the left subclavian artery, where the position is confirmed by fluoroscopy. Observation of the central arterial pressure tracing allows timing of balloon inflation to occur at the onset of diastole, indicated by the dicrotic notch (Fig. 3.4). Deflation should occur before the aortic valve opens to allow forward flow of blood with minimal afterload. The time of deflation is chosen to give the greatest drop in end-diastolic pressure, usually 5 to 15 mmHg. The effects of inflation and deflation timing errors on the arterial wave form are shown in Figure 3.5. After the timing has been set, the balloon cycle can be triggered either by the electrocardiogram or arterial pressure tracing.

Patients in whom major ischemia is unlikely but evidence of severe hypoperfusion persists despite aggressive drug therapy should be considered for placement of ventricular assist or total artificial devices. Patients with an intraaortic balloon who do not show major improvement within the first hours should also be considered for other devices. Before inserting a support device of any type, it should be decided whether the patient would be a candidate for transplantation if his condition stabilizes. Those who would not be a candidate under any circumstances should rarely be given an assist device, as weaning is seldom possible if the device was clearly necessary at the time of insertion. Spontaneous recovery allowing device removal is more likely in patients after cardiopulmonary bypass than in patients with more chronic conditions.

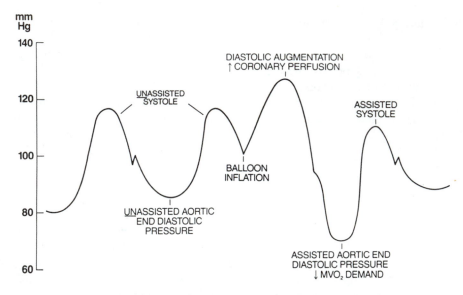

FIGURE 3.4. Idealized central arterial waveforms during unassisted systole and during a cycle assisted by intraaortic balloon counterpulsation. Illustration courtesy of Datascope Corp.

Therapy of Unstable Patients

After the tailoring of total afterload reduction, approximately 90% of patients can initially be stabilized after referral with severe symptoms of heart failure. Within the first month after discharge, out-patients are evaluated for maintained stability (Table 3.3), present in about two-thirds of those initially stabilized (Fig. 3.2). However, one-third of the initially stabilized patients cannot maintain stable renal function, serum sodium, blood pressure, absence of symptomatic arrhythmias, or frequent angina. Whether or not these patients are hospitalized or out-patients frequently depends on the community, out-patient, and in-patient resources of the center rather than on patient status.

The best management strategy for such patients remains in question. Intermittent infusions of inotropic agents may be of some use, primarily for promoting diuresis.[33] Out-patient inotropic infusions may allow patients to remain at home,[34] but have been associated with increased mortality when used in high doses. Oral therapy with experimental phosphodiesterase inhibitors may improve short-term status, but most studies have addressed their effects in more stable patients, in whom life span has not been prolonged. As renal function is frequently the limiting factor, intermittent dialysis may play a role in maintaining these patients in a comfortable fluid balance without excessive levels of blood urea nitro-

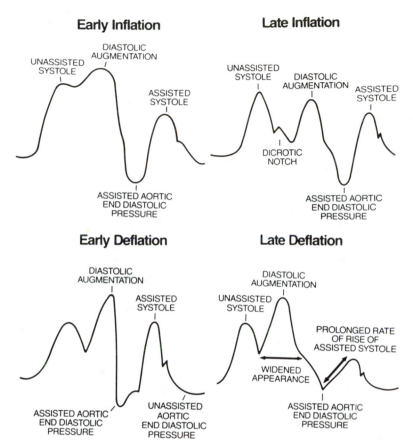

FIGURE 3.5. Central arterial waveforms demonstrating the timing errors of early and late inflation and deflation of the intraaortic balloon. Illustration courtesy of Datascope Corp.

TABLE 3.3. Outpatient stability on tailored therapy.

Stable weight on oral diuretics
Stable creatinine (usually ≤2.0 mg/dl)
Stable blood urea nitrogen (usually ≤60 mg/dl)
Stable serum sodium (usually ≥130 mEq/L)
Absence of frequent angina
Absence of symptomatic arrhythmias (other than sensed PVCs[a])
Ambulatory status ≥1 city block

[a]PVC = premature ventricular contraction.

gen,[35] but has not been systematically investigated in this particular population.

The unstable patient is at high risk for sudden death, which may result from many mechanisms. Avoidable secondary factors such as hyperkalemia[36] and hypokalemia, hypomagnesemia, and excessive antiarrhythmic drug levels should be carefully monitored in these patients with fluctuating hepatic and renal clearances.

Related Risks in Heart Failure

The major risk for both stable and unstable out-patients with heart failure is sudden death, defined as occurring without warning or during sleep. In patients followed on tailored therapy, in whom re-hospitalization or expeditious transplantation can be considered, sudden death accounts for more than 80% of all deaths, compared to 30% to 50% in heart failure patients with varying therapeutics and varying availability for vigilant follow-up.[37]

It had previously been assumed that most of these deaths resulted from ventricular tachyarrhythmias, a plausible assumption based on the presence of nonsustained ventricular arrhythmias in up to 80% of patients with advanced heart failure, and on the evidence regarding inducibility of ventricular tachycardia in survivors of sudden death without heart failure. However, sudden death in heart failure patients has not been able to be predicted by electrophysiologic study[38] and has not been shown to be prevented by amiodarone.[39] The failure of these approaches to decrease sudden death may reflect the frequency of sudden death due to causes other than primary ventricular tachyarrhythmias. Monitored arrests in patients with stable heart failure have frequently resulted from primary bradycardic rhythms,[40] perhaps due to abnormal intracardiac reflexes. Fatal cardiac arrests in heart failure can also result from emboli to lungs, brain, or coronary arteries.[40,41] Whereas patients with coronary artery disease are more likely than patients with nonischemic cardiomyopathy to have primary ventricular tachyarrhythmias,[40] recurrent infarction is frequently their cause of death.

Our current approach to the management of arrhythmias is to treat atrial arrhythmias and symptomatic ventricular arrhythmias (arrhythmias associated with discomfort, hemodynamic compromise, or syncope) with procainamide, quinidine, or amiodarone. Therapy with mexilitine is employed occasionally for ventricular arrhythmias but is frequently limited by side effects. Type 1C agents such as flecainide frequently depress ventricular function and are associated with a higher incidence of proarrhythmic effects in patients with low ejection fractions. Patients in our program are not treated for asymptomatic nonsustained ventricular tachycardia unless episodes are very frequent or exceed 180 beats/min.

Patients with dilated ventricles are at increased risk for embolic events that occur silently or can cause disability, ineligibility for transplantation, or death. Emboli may originate from the atria or ventricles, and from the systemic venous system particularly when mobility is limited. The frequency of embolic events has not been established prospectively for a large, unselected population of heart failure patients. However, 10% to 20% of patients with dilated cardiomyopathy have developed clinical emboli during their course[42,43] for an estimated incidence of three to four events per 100 patient years. Patients dying with cardiomyopathy have evidence of emboli in up to 60% of cases, one-half of which were clinically evident.[44] Whereas echocardiographic characterization of ventricular thrombi in living patients did not predict subsequent embolic events,[43] pathologic identification of both ventricular and atrial mural thrombi and plaques did correlate with the presence of emboli at necropsy.[41]

Retrospective data indicate that the incidence of embolization is reduced by anticoagulation with warfarin derivatives.[41] Although the optimal degree of anticoagulation is not known, patients with fluctuating hepatic congestion and function are at particular risk for hemorrhagic complications. There are currently two strategies for anticoagulation in patients with dilated ventricular failure. One strategy is to anticoagulate all patients, including those awaiting transplantation (at which time vitamin K is given parenterally). The other strategy is to anticoagulate only those who may be at particularly high risk. Whereas left ventricular thrombi and atrial fibrillation appear to be risk factors in some studies but not in others, bed rest and history of previous embolic events may be the biggest risk factors for future embolic events. Careful supervision, particularly for hepatic congestion, and a limited goal of 16 to 18 sec for the protime may minimize hemorrhagic risk in this population.

Waiting List Expectation and Priority

As waiting lists grow and the waiting times lengthen, decisions during the waiting period are becoming increasingly important. The current list for hearts in the United States is more than 1500 patients long, with 50% more patients added than transplanted each month. The current waiting time on the national list is longer than 5 months.[2]

Decisions regarding recipient priority should reflect the goal of maximizing survival for the heart failure population, not survival for the transplanted hearts. Re-evaluation of patients after tailored therapy allows distribution to maximize survival benefit, as shown in the Shoulder curves of survival with heart failure (Fig. 3.6). The 10% of eligible patients with persistent critical status have a postoperative mortality that is more than twice that of stable out-patients, but 1-year survival still approaches 80% for critical patients, who otherwise would not survive.[44] These patients

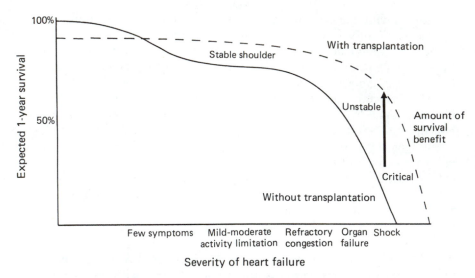

FIGURE 3.6. The Shoulder curves of estimated survival with and without cardiac transplantation for patients according to the clinical severity of heart failure. With progressive hemodynamic compromise, the absolute survival declines slightly but the relative survival benefit of transplantation increases greatly.

have a greater expected benefit in terms of improved life expectancy than patients who can be stabilized on medical therapy, who may have up to 70% 1-year survival without transplantation, the major mortality being from sudden death. The 30% of patients who are unstable have a limited quality of life and life span, tend to have frequent hospital readmissions, and should receive higher priority than stable out-patients.

The quality of life is frequently not severely limited for the 60% of patients stabilized on tailored therapy, many of whom will wish to defer or avoid transplantation, although the survival may be improved by transplantation. Exercise capacity and quality of life at least in one study was similar for sustained medical therapy versus cardiac transplantation, which would therefore be performed primarily to prolong life in this population.[45] When better understanding of the mechanisms of sudden death has improved our ability to predict or prevent it, decisions regarding transplantation in hemodynamically stable patients will be easier.

As patients spend more time on the transplant list, their priority is raised, in harmony with the philosophy of "Stand in line and wait your turn". However, it has long been observed that most deaths in heart failure occur in the first few months after referral.[38] Among patients eligible for cardiac transplantation, the greatest jeopardy occurs in the first 6 months after evaluation, after which mortality over the next 12 months is similar whether transplantation is performed or not.[46] Thus, patients who remain stable after 6 months on the waiting list may merit re-evaluation as candidates at that time, rather than automatic promotion to higher priority.

Conclusions

Cardiac transplantation is a glamorous and effective therapy but the donor shortage limits transplantation to a minority of patients with advanced heart failure, who may expect long waiting periods even if accepted. It is essential that all patients referred undergo systematic tailoring of medical therapy not only to minimize the number of urgent transplants and improve waiting list status, but also to offer the best chance for improved quality and length of life to the entire population with advanced heart failure.

References

1. Evans RW, Mannihen DL, Garrison LP, Maier AM. Donor availability as the primary determinant of the future of heart transplantation. *JAMA.* 1986;255:1892–1898.
2. United Network of Organ Sharing Update 1988;4:1–11.
3. Cohn JN, Veterans Administration Cooperative. Effect of vasodilator therapy on mortality in chronic congestive heart failure. *N Engl J Med.* 1986;314:1547–1552.
4. Pfeffer MA, Pfeffer JM, Skinberg C, Finn P. Survival after an experimental myocardial infarction: beneficial effects of long-term therapy with captopril. *Circulation.* 1985;72:406–413.
5. Feldman AM, Cates AE, Baumgartner W, Baugham KL, Van Dop C. Alterations of the Mr 40,000 pertussis toxin substrate in human heart failure. *Circulation.* 1987;76:IV–432.
6. Fowler MB, Laser JA, Hopkins GL, Minobe W, Bristow MR. Assessment of the beta-adrenergic receptor pathway in the intact failing human heart: progressive receptor down-regulation and subsensitivity to agonist response. *Circulation.* 1986;74:1290–1302.
7. Klein HH, Spaar U, Schlepple, Wiegand V, Kreuzer H. Comparative analysis of myocardial enzyme activities of the energy-supplying metabolism in patients with dilative cardiomyopathies and valve diseases. *Clin Cardiol.* 1986;9:197–202.
8. Weisman HF, Weisfeldt ML. Toward an understanding of the molecular basis of cardiomyopathies. *J Am Coll Cardiol.* 1987;11:1135–1138.
9. Feldman MD, Copelas L, Gwathmey JK, et al. Deficient production of cyclic AMP; pharmacologic evidence of an important cause of contractile dysfunction in patients with end-stage heart failure. *Circulation.* 1987;7:331–339.
10. Strauss RH, Stevenson LW, Dadourian BJ, Child JS. The predictability of mitral regurgitation detected by Doppler echocardiography in patients referred for cardiac transplantation. *Am J Cardiol.* 1987;59:892–894.
11. Lang RM, Borow KM, Neumann A, Janzen D. Systemic vascular resistance: an unreliable index of left ventricular afterload. *Circulation.* 1986;74:1114–1123.

12. Carr JG, Stevenson LW, Walden JA, Heber D. Prevalence and hemodynamic correlates of malnutrition in severe congestive heart failure secondary to ischemic or idiopathic dilated cardiomyopathy. *Am J Cardiol*. 1989;63:709–713.

13. Greenberg TT, Richmond WH, Stocking RA, Gupta PD, Meehan JP, Henry JP. Impaired atrial receptor responses in dogs with heart failure due to tricuspid insufficiency and pulmonary artery stenosis. *Circ Res*. 1973;32:424–433.

14. Leimbach WN, Wallin BG, Victor RG, Aylward PE, Sundlof G, Mark AL. Direct evidence from intraneural recordings for increased central sympathetic outflow in patients with heart failure. *Circulation*. 1986;73:913–919.

15. Dzau VJ. Vascular renin-angiotensin system in hypertension: new insights into the mechanism of action of angiotensin-converting enzyme inhibitors. *Am J Med*. 1988;84:4–12A.

16. Goldsmith SR, Francis GS, Cowley AW, Goldenberg IF, Cohn JN. Hemodynamic effects of infused arginine vasopressin in congestive heart failure. *J Am Coll Cardiol*. 1986;8:779–83.

17. Wilkins MR, Stott RAW, Lewis HM. Atrial natriuretic factor. *Ann Clin Biochem*. 1989;26:115–118.

18. Cohn JN, Levine TB, Olivari MT, et al. Plasma norepinephrine as a guide to prognosis in patients with chronic congestive heart failure. *N Engl J Med*. 1984;311:819–823.

19. Lee WH, Packer M. Prognostic importance of serum sodium concentration and its modification by converting-enzyme inhibition in patients with severe chronic heart failure. *Circulation*. 1986;73:257–267.

20. Hamilton M, Stevenson LW, Luu M, Stevenson WG, Walden J. Abnormal tri-iodothyronine is the strongest short-term prognostic factor identified in advanced heart failure. *J Am Coll Cardiol*. 1990;65:1209–1212.

21. Unverferth DV, Magorien RD, Moeschberger ML, Baker PB, Fetters JK, Leier CV. Factors influencing the one-year mortality of dilated cardiomyopathy. *Am J Cardiol*. 1984;54:147–152.

22. Franciosa JA, Wilen M, Ziesche S, Cohn JN. Survival in men with severe chronic left ventricular failure due to either coronary heart disease or idiopathic dilated cardiomyopathy. *Am J Cardiol*. 1983;51:831–836.

23. Stevenson LW, Dracup KA, Tillisch JH. The efficacy of medical therapy tailored for severe congestive heart failure in patients transferred for urgent transplantation. *Am J Cardiol*. 1989;63:461–464.

24. Stevenson LW, Perloff JK. The limited reliability of physical signs for estimating hemodynamics in chronic heart failure. *JAMA*. 1989;261:884–888.

25. Stevenson LW, Tillisch JH. Maintenance of cardiac output with normal filling pressures in dilated heart failure. *Circulation*. 1986;74:1303–1308.

26. Stevenson LW, Belil D, Grover-McKay M, et al. Effects of afterload reduction on left ventricular volume and mitral regurgitation in severe congestive heart failure. *Am J Cardiol*. 1987;60:654–658.

27. Marone C, Muggle F, Lahn W, Frey FJ. Pharmacokinetic and pharmacodynamic interaction between furosemide and metolazone in man. *Eur J Clin Invest*. 1985;15:253–257.

28. Hershberger RE, Bristow MR. Receptor alterations in the failing human heart. *Heart Fail*. 1988;6:230–238.

29. Franciosa JA. Intravenous amrinone: an advance or a wrong step? *Ann Intern Med*. 1985;102:399–400. Editorial.

30. Bouvier M, Collins S, Campbell P, O'Dowd B, Caron MG, Lefkowitz RJ. Two distinct pathways for cAMP-receptor mediated down-regulation of the beta-2 adrenergic receptor: Phosphorylation of the receptor and regulation of its mRNA level. *Clin Res.* 1989;37:531A.

31. Dunkman WB, Leinbach RC, Buckley MJ, et al. Clinical and hemodynamic results of intraaortic balloon pumping and surgery for cardiogenic shock. *Circulation.* 1972;46:465–477.

32. Pierri MK, Zema M, Kligfield P, et al. Exercise tolerance in late survivors of balloon pumping and surgery for cardiogenic shock. *Circulation.* 1980;62:I138–I141.

33. Leier CV, Huss RN, Lewis RP, Unverferth DV. Drug-induced conditioning in congestive heart failure. *Circulation.* 1982;65:1382–1387.

34. Miller LW. Ambulatory inotropic therapy as a bridge to cardiac transplantation. *J Am Coll Cardiol.* 1987;9:89A.

35. DiLeo M, Pacitti A, Bergerone S, et al. Ultrafiltration in the treatment of refractory congestive heart failure. *Clin Cardiol.* 1988;11:449–452.

36. Chakko SC, Frutchey J, Gheorghiade M. Life-threatening hyperkalemia in severe heart failure. *Am Heart J.* 1989;117:1083–1091.

37. Wilson JR, Schwartz JS, St. John Sutton M, et al. Prognosis in severe heart failure: relation to hemodynamic measurements and ventricular ectopic activity. *J Am Coll Cardiol* 1983;2:403–409.

38. Stevenson WG, Stevenson LW, Weiss J, Tillisch JH. Programmed ventricular stimulation in severe heart failure: high, short-term risk of sudden death despite noninducibility. *Am Heart J.* 1988;116:1447–1454.

39. Nicklas JM, Mickelson JK, Das SK, Morady F, Schork MA, Pitt B. Prospective randomized double-blind placebo-controlled trial of low-dose amiodarone in patients with severe heart failure and frequent ventricular ectopy. *Circulation.* 1988;78:II–29. Abstract.

40. Luu M, Stevenson WG, Stevenson LW, Baron K, Walden JA. Diverse mechanisms of unexpected sudden death in heart failure. *Circulation.* 1989;80:1075–1080.

41. Roberts WC, Siegel RJ, McManus BM. Idiopathic dilated cardiomyopathy: analysis of 152 necropsy patients. *Am J Cardiol.* 1987;60:1340–1355.

42. Fuster V, Gersh BJ, Guiliani ER, Tajik AJ, Brandenburg RO, Frye RL. The natural history of dilated cardiomyopathy. *Am J Cardiol.* 1981;47:525–531.

43. Gottdeiner JS, Gay JA, VanVoorhees L, DiBianco R, Fletcher RD. Frequency and embolic potential of left ventricular thrombus in dilated cardiomyopathy: assessment by 2-dimensional echocardiography. *Am J Cardiol.* 1983;52:1281–1285.

44. Stevenson LW, Donohue BC, Tillisch JH, et al. Urgent priority transplantation: when should it be done? *J Heart Transplant.* 1987;6:267–272.

45. Stevenson LW, Sietsema K, Tillisch JH, et al. Exercise capacity for survivors of cardiac transplantation or sustained medical therapy for stable heart failure. *Circulation.* 1990;81:78–85.

46. Stevenson LW, Moriguchi JD, Kobashigawa JA, et al. Decreasing survival benefit of cardiac transplantation as waiting list lengthens. *Circulation.* 1989;80:II–671.

4
Ventricular Assistance as a Bridge to Cardiac Transplantation

D. GLEN PENNINGTON AND MARC T. SWARTZ

Over the last 10 years there has been increasing success in the field of cardiac transplantation. Improvements in survival and life style along with the more widespread use of cardiac transplantation is well documented in this book. However, continued growth in the field of cardiac transplantation is limited by several factors, the primary factor being the scarcity of donor organs.[1] Over the same 10-year period, dramatic advances have been made in the field of mechanical circulatory support. Cardiac transplantation and mechanical circulatory support have recently merged to offer a significant percentage of high-risk patients the possibility of being bridged to cardiac transplantation.[2-5] The development of cyclosporine therapy and advancements in the efficiency of circulatory support devices have made this combination a realistic option for some patients who would otherwise die.

The first attempts to bridge patients to cardiac transplantation occurred 20 years ago at the Texas Heart Institute.[6,7] Unfortunately, these patients developed common complications, infection, and multiple organ failure. There were also significant problems with the devices. Since these initial attempts, there have been improvements in the efficiency and fit of the devices, patient selection, and patient management.

Owing to the complexity of the problems associated with the use of total artificial hearts (TAH) and ventricular assist devices (VAD), several centers have tried less complicated devices to bridge patients to transplantation. The period from 1978 to 1984 was marked by attempts by several different groups to use intraaortic balloon pumps (IABP) and extracorporeal membrane oxygenation (ECMO) before cardiac transplantation.[8,9] The initial success of Reemstma and associates in supporting three patients with an IABP before cardiac transplantation are the first documented successful cases of bridging patients to cardiac transplantation with a mechanical assist device. The success of the IABP has been further documented by the achievements of the University of Pittsburgh group.[10] Therefore, the IABP currently represents the preferred initial technique in treatment of patients who develop cardiogenic shock

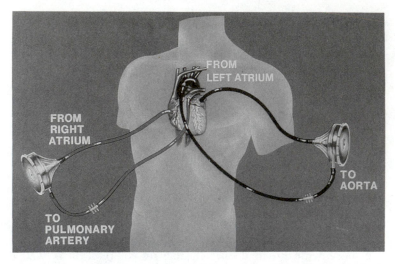

FIGURE 4.1. Biventricular support with Biomedicus centrifugal pumps showing atrial cannulation.

while awaiting cardiac transplantation. Venoarterial ECMO before cardiac transplantation was described by Pennington and associates at St. Louis University.[11] The use of ECMO in cardiac transplant recipients has been limited in comparison to other methods because of the significant complications related to current ECMO systems.

The period from September 1984 to September 1985 was marked by the first successful clinical applications of bridging to transplantation with an implantable left ventricular assist system (LVAS),[12] an external heterotopic pulsatile VAD,[13] and a TAH.[14] Subsequent bridging experiences have employed a variety of circulatory support devices with a moderate degree of success and have made this therapeutic option a growing and important part of many cardiac transplantation programs.

Description of Devices and Techniques of Insertion

Centrifugal Pumps

Centrifugal pumps developed and manufactured by Biomedicus, Inc. (Eden Prairie, MN) (Fig. 4.1) and Sarns, Inc. (Ann Arbor, MI) have been used to bridge patients to transplantation.[5] Centrifugal pumps use rotating cones or impellers to generate energy that is recovered in the form of pressure-flow work. While operating at a constant speed, the pumps generate nearly constant pressure over a wide range of flow rates. The pumping action is transmitted by magnetic coupling to the mated drive magnet. Currrently, there are no specific cannulae designed for centrifu-

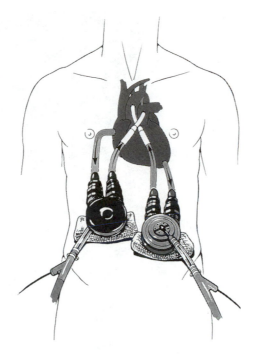

FIGURE 4.2. Pierce-Donachy Thoratec biventricular assist devices.

gal pumps; however, most investigators have been able to contrive systems using standard cardiopulmonary bypass cannulae and tubing. The
insertion of centrifugal pumps currently requires a sternotomy and if the
patient is unstable, placement on standard cardiopulmonary bypass.
Pursestring sutures can be placed in the right or left atrium for insertion
of the atrial cannula. A standard aortic cannula can be placed through
a pursestring suture into the ascending aorta or the main pulmonary
artery for return of flow. For left-sided support, withdrawal cannulae
can also be placed in the left ventricular apex with return to the ascending
aorta.

External Pulsatile Ventricular Assist Devices

External pulsatile VADs such as the Thoratec (Fig. 4.2) and Symbion
(Fig. 4.3) are constructed of a rigid housing and contain a flexible sac or
diaphragm. These devices use mechanical inlet and outlet valves. Pump
inlet cannulae are available for the atria or left ventricular apex with the
Thoratec system and atria for the Symbion Acute Ventricular Assist Device (AVAD). The Abiomed (Fig. 4.4) pump differs from the Thoratec
and the Symbion AVAD in that it uses polyurethane valves. It can be

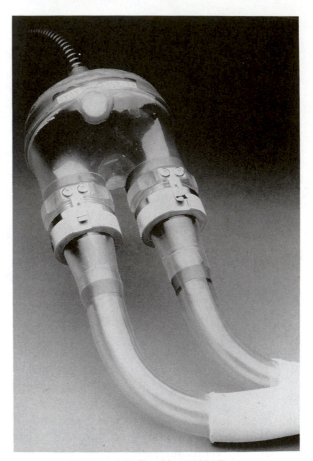

FIGURE 4.3. Symbion AVAD.

used only for atrial cannulation—left ventricular apex cannulation is not an option. The Dacron graft on the polyurethane outflow cannula of all systems in this group may be sutured to the aorta or the pulmonary artery depending on whether left or right ventricular support is required. If atrial cannulation is used, a venous drainage cannula shaped to a right angle can be placed in either atrium with a simple pursestring suture around the atrial appendage. It is also possible to place the atrial cannula through a pursestring suture near the entrance of the right superior pulmonary vein into the left atrium. Left ventricular cannulation is more complex and requires removal of a portion of the left ventricle. The left ventricular apex cannula is secured using multiple sutures through a sewing ring located on the cannula.[15]

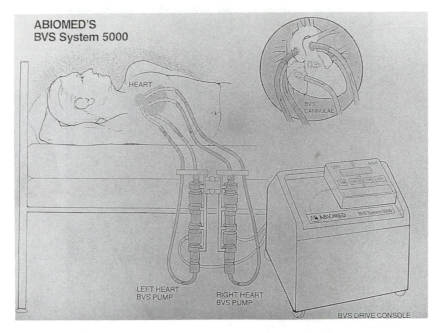

ABIOMED'S
BVS System 5000

HEART

BVS
CANNULAE

LEFT HEART
BVS PUMP

RIGHT HEART
BVS PUMP

BVS DRIVE CONSOLE

FIGURE 4.4. Abiomed BVS.

Implantable Left Ventricular Assist Devices

Currently, the National Heart, Lung and Blood Institute is sponsoring the development of permanent, implantable LVASs. All of the components of these systems, which will allow them to be completely implanted, are not yet available. However, excellent pumps have been developed and are in clinical use. Currently, these pumps are used with externalized energy sources to bridge patients to transplantation. These devices are heterotopic in position and the pump is implanted in the abdomen.[16] Pump inflow involves cannulation of the left ventricular apex and pump outflow is through a graft sutured to the ascending aorta. Full cardiopulmonary bypass is required for insertion of these devices.

Total Artificial Heart

The Jarvik-7 TAH (Fig. 4.5) has been the most commonly used device for bridging to cardiac transplantation. The Jarvik TAH is an orthotopic biventricular replacement device whose implantation is similar to a cardiac transplant.[17] Connections to the natural atria are made with a quick-connect system using polyurethane atrial cuffs. Dacron grafts are sewn

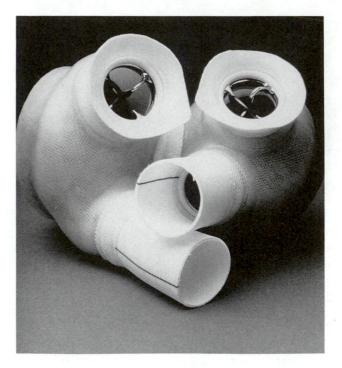

FIGURE 4.5. Jarvik-7-70 TAH.

to the aorta and pulmonary artery. A smaller model, the Jarvik-7-70, can be implanted in smaller patients, but it has also been used in larger patients at higher pumping rates.

Patient Selection

It is imperative that patient selection criteria be developed that will allow the survival rate of patients bridged to transplantation to be comparable to those receiving conventional transplantation. Patients being considered for assist devices should have maximal drug therapy, treatment of acid-base imbalance, correction of hypoxemia, and volume replacement. The initial choice of mechanical support should be an IABP, except in patients with severe peripheral vascular disease, which may be considered a contraindication to cardiac transplantation. Hemodynamic criteria for considering patients for mechanical circulatory support are well established: cardiac output index <1.8 L/m^2 per min; left and/or right atrial pressure >20 mmHg; urine output <20 cc/hr (adult); elevated systemic vascular resistance; other evidence of decreasing peripheral perfusion, such as cool extremities, acidosis, or decreased sensorium. Patients who meet these criteria will probably not survive if allowed to remain in this condition. Most patients have a history of chronic illness and gradual decompensation. However, there are patients who deteriorate abruptly. Some patients who have already been selected as heart transplant recipients deteriorate suddenly while awaiting a donor heart. These patients probably represent the best patient group, since much of their past history is readily available. Additionally, the transplant team is familiar with these patients and has often managed their medical therapy for some period of time.

Patients with postcardiotomy cardiogenic shock have been the most widely studied group in relation to circulatory assist devices.[18-20] Evidence of myocardial recovery in our series of postcardiotomy patients has been as high as 50% despite the fact that the overall survival rate is less.[21] There have been extensive efforts to determine which postcardiotomy patients might be expected to recover myocardial function. One factor leading to a negative outcome has been the occurrence of an acute perioperative myocardial infarction.[22] Another predictor of nonsurvival has been the presence of biventricular failure.[23] If biventricular support is required, the assist methods become more complicated and the probability of survival in the recovery group diminishes. This increased mortality is influenced by the fact that perioperative myocardial infarctions often involve both the left and right ventricle. The presence of an acute perioperative myocardial infarction and biventricular failure is a combination that strongly mitigates against myocardial recovery and is justification for transplantation. If properly supported, biventricular failure should not be a negative determinant of survival in the bridge-to-transplant population since myocardial recovery is not an issue.

Acute myocardial infarction shock patients are another potential group. This group may have an increased chance for survival because they have not had a chronic illness that left them debilitated. If the initial period of cardiogenic shock can be reversed by medical therapy or circulatory assistance, these patients will probably make excellent cardiac transplant recipients. However, they are often admitted to the emergency room, intensive care unit, or cardiac catheterization laboratory with acute massive infarctions and cardiogenic shock. In these patients, it may be beneficial to support them with femorofemoral ECMO until cardiac catheterization and other diagnostic studies can be performed in order to determine if they are transplant candidates. If so, they should undergo placement of a more sophisticated device within 24 hours of initiation of ECMO.

Our philosophy is that a strong contraindication to cardiac transplantation, such as renal failure requiring dialysis, uncontrollable sepsis, or age over 65 years would also be a contraindication to the institution of circulatory support. Other conditions such as severe coagulopathy, cerebral injury, or liver failure must also be considered contraindications to

TABLE 4.1. Selection of devices.

ECMO	Resuscitation/stabilization
	Ventricular failure with severe pulmonary insufficiency
	Patients too small for other devices
External VAD	Reversible failure (L, R or BV[a])
	Isolated LV[b] failure (too small for LVAS)—Tx[c] candidate
	Irreversible failure (L, R, or BV)—Tx candidate
LVAS	Isolated irreversible LV failure–Tx candidate
TAH	Irreversible BV failure—Tx candidate
	Irreversible failure—clots in heart—Tx candidate

[a]BV = biventricular.
[b]LV = left ventricular.
[c]Tx = transplant.

both mechanical circulatory support and cardiac transplantation. Only the best candidates should be selected in order to assure that no donor organs are wasted.

Type of Support Required

The diagnosis of left, right, or biventricular failure is important in determining what type of mechanical support device should be used. Early investigators believed that mechanical support of the left ventricle was essential and that inotropic drugs could be used to treat right ventricular failure.[24–26] Often, severe biventricular failure may not be recognized early in the course of mechanical assistance. Biventricular assist devices (BVAD) have now been applied successfully in the bridge-to-transplant patients with good results.[2] A recent study demonstrated that approximately 60% of those patients being bridged to cardiac transplantation have biventricular failure. Isolated left ventricular failure occurs approximately 40% of the time and isolated right ventricular failure is rare.[27] The etiology of heart failure has not been useful in determining the need for biventricular support. In general, the atrium with the highest pressure indicates the ventricle with predominant failure. In most instances, left ventricular support is initiated first and this may unmask failure of the right ventricle, necessitating insertion of a right ventricular assist device (RVAD). Our criteria for our selection of devices are outlined in Table 4.1. If there is severe biventricular dysfunction in a patient who has already been selected for cardiac transplantation, a TAH or BVADs may be appropriate. However, if there is severe left ventricular dysfunction and satisfactory right ventricular function, a left ventricular assist device (LVAD) should be used.

TABLE 4.2. Results of bridging to transplantation.

Device	# Patients	# Tx[a]	# Survived	% Survival after Tx	Longest successful perfusion (days)
Centrifugal	35	22	15	68	30
Thoratec	84	59	47	80	81
Symbion AVAD	61[b]	7	5	71	65
Abiomed	43[b]	20	8	40	19
Novacor	13	15	13	87	91
Thermedics	12	7	3	43	40
Jarvik-7 TAH	142	102	74	73	34

[a]Tx = transplant.
[b]Includes postcardiotomy and bridge-to-transplant patients.

Clinical Experience

Since 1984 there has been widespread interest in using mechanical support devices to bridge patients to cardiac transplantation. The development of new systems and the greater availability of devices have allowed wider application of these techniques. The information presented in this chapter is derived from various sources including communications from investigators, manufacturers and the combined registry for mechanical assist devices and artificial hearts of the American Society of Artificial Internal Organs (ASAIO) and the International Society of Heart Transplantation (ISHT), which is maintained at Pennsylvania State University. Since this is a voluntary registry not all of the cases have been reported. Also, there are no uniform criteria to define complications and survival. Therefore, any comparisons between devices in this chapter must be kept in perspective. The results of bridge to transplantation with the currently used devices are presented in Table 4.2.

Thirty-five patients were supported with centrifugal pumps as a bridge to cardiac transplantation. Twenty-two of these 35 patients were actually transplanted with 15 long-term survivors. The 68% survival rate after transplantation is comparable to other devices currently being used in the same capacity. One patient was supported at the Cleveland Clinic for 30 days with a centrifugal pump before successful cardiac transplantation.[28] This represents the longest successful bridge-to-transplant perfusion with a centrifugal device. Most of the centrifugal pump patients were transplanted within 7 days, emphasizing the importance of obtaining donor hearts early in the course of circulatory support with these patients. The limitations of centrifugal pumps have been the necessity to maintain continuous anticoagulation with heparin, a slightly higher rate of hemolysis, and the lack of ability to mobilize patients and get them out of bed.

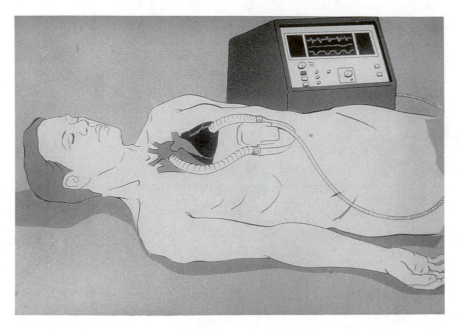

FIGURE 4.6. Novacor LVAS.

External pulsatile VADs have also been used successfully in a significant number of patients before cardiac transplantation. Eighty-four patients were supported with a Thoratec VAD, of whom 59 were transplanted and 47 survived. The impressive survival rate of those patients who actually underwent cardiac transplantation (80%) demonstrates the efficiency of this pump. The main advantages of this type of device are its multiple cannulation options and the ability to provide biventricular support if necessary. Successful perfusions have been obtained for as long as 81 days, documenting the capability of this type of device to support patients for 2 to 3 months. The Symbion AVAD is a newer device that has been used in at least seven patients as a bridge to transplantation. Five patients survived transplantation; the longest perfusion was 65 days.

The Abiomed biventricular support (BVS) is a pneumatic extracorporeal system that has been used in at least 20 patients who received transplants. Eight of these patients survived (40%).

Implantable LVASs such as the Novacor (Fig. 4.6) and Thermedics (Fig. 4.7) have been used in 45 patients as a bridge to cardiac transplantation. Twenty-two patients were transplanted, with 16 survivors. The overall survival rate was 87% for Novacor patients and 43% for the Thermedics patients. Both of these systems are prototypes of permanent systems and can be used to support patients for several months.

To date, the only survivors of transplantation after support with a TAH

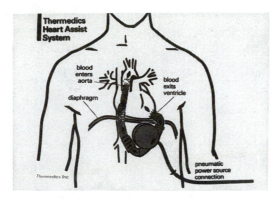

FIGURE 4.7. Thermedics left heart assist system.

have been patients who received the Jarvik device manufactured by Symbion Corporation (Tempe, AZ). One hundred forty-two patients have received 145 devices. Three patients received a second TAH after rejecting their first transplant. The length of time on Jarvik-7 TAH before transplantation ranged from 1 to 244 days, with a median time of 9 days. One hundred two patients received transplants, of whom 74 survived 30 days. This 73% survival of patients transplanted is impressive; however, in this group of patients a considerable number died within a few months of transplantation. Of the first 100 patients to receive the Jarvik device as a bridge to cardiac transplantation, the "long-term" survival rate after transplantation was 54%.[29]

Complications were common in this critically ill group of patients awaiting transplantation. Table 4.3 shows the complications associated with bridging to transplantation with VADs. These data were obtained from the ASAIO-ISHT registry. Bleeding was the most common complication, occurring in 40% of all patients. Fifty-six percent of those patients who died had bleeding complications as opposed to 25% of the survivors.

TABLE 4.3. Complications associated with ventricular assist devices[a] bridge to transplantation.

	Incidence		
Complication	Total patients (%) (N = 134)	Survived (%) (N = 68)	Died (%) (N = 66)
Bleeding/reoperate	40	25	56
Renal failure	16	0	33
Biventricular failure	22	16	33
Infection	16	10	21
Embolus	4	1	5

[a]Data from ASAIO-ISHT Registry.

TABLE 4.4. Complications associated with total artificial hearts[a] bridge to transplantation.

	Incidence		
Complications	Total patients (%) (N = 82)	Survived (%) (N = 38)	Died (%) (N = 44)
Bleeding/reoperate	44	32	55
Renal failure	29	8	48
Infection	32	21	41
Embolus	17	18	16

[a]Data from ASAIO-ISHT Registry.

Another significant factor affecting survival in bridge-to-transplant patients was renal failure. Sixteen percent of patients with VADs suffered from renal failure, all of whom died. Twenty-two percent of the patients who were bridged with VADs had biventricular failure. The incidence of biventricular failure was twice as high in those who died as opposed to those who survived, suggesting, perhaps, that a considerable number of patients had biventricular failure that was inadequately treated. Sixteen percent of the patients suffered infectious complications, with an incidence ratio in those who died versus those who survived of 2 : 1. Since the development of cyclosporine and improvements in immunosuppressive regimens, infectious complications after bridge-to-transplantation procedures have been less than was previously feared. Four percent of the overall patient population suffered an embolic event—1% of those who survived versus 5% of those who died. This is a low thromboembolic rate, considering that some patients were supported for more than two weeks. Initially, many believed that a much higher percentage of patients would suffer thromboembolism.

Complications associated with bridging to transplantation with TAHs is located in Table 4.4. Overall complication rates were higher in the TAH group compared to the VAD group. Again, bleeding, renal failure, and infection were the major complications encountered. As with the VAD group, renal failure was much more prevalent in the nonsurvivors than the survivors. Bleeding and infection also significantly affected patient outcome. Biventricular failure was obviously not a complication in patients with a TAH. Thromboembolic events were more common in the TAH group compared to the VAD group. Seventeen percent of the total TAH group suffered embolic events as opposed to 4% of the VAD group.

Discussion

It is apparent from the above description that bridging to transplantation with circulatory support devices has been quite successful, with salvage rates much higher than in patients receiving VADs for myocardial recovery. In the better series, such as the Thoratec and Novacor, the chance for survival in patients who are transplanted is almost as good as in the routine cardiac transplant population. However, in this era of increased competition for a limited donor supply, efforts must be continued to improve the results with bridging devices. The rewards of these efforts will not only be better results for the small number of bridged patients, but will enormously impact on our ultimate application of permanent systems. Therefore, it is important to assess carefully those factors that determine success.

Selection of the appropriate device and cannulation techniques are important factors to consider. Mild to moderate right ventricular failure usually can be managed with drugs, but not many patients develop severe right ventricular failure, which is unresponsive to inotropic drugs. In these patients, biventricular support must be used. If right ventricular function is in question, it is preferable to use a device with the capability of biventricular support, insert the LVAD first and use inotropic support for the right ventricle. If the LVAD does not fill adequately despite elevated right atrial pressures, a RVAD should be inserted. Vigorous pharmacological therapy is appropriate before RVAD insertion, but it should not prolong the period of hypoperfusion and jeopardize vital organ function.

From the descriptions of the various devices, it is apparent that centrifugal and external pulsatile pumps can be used for right and left ventricular support, and can be used in either the atria or the left ventricle. The implantable LVAS devices must be placed in the left ventricular apex, and therefore are not useful for right ventricular support. If a LVAS is used, patients with predominantly left ventricular failure should be selected. If right ventricular failure occurs, it must be treated with pharmacological therapy or another device that can provide right ventricular support. In postcardiotomy or myocardial infarction patients, it is advantageous to use left atrial cannulation because it avoids further destruction of myocardial tissue. Left atrial cannulation is not important in potential heart transplant recipients. Therefore, if there is no consideration of myocardial recovery, left ventricular apex cannulation is preferred.

The more sophisticated systems require insertion in the operating room with full cardiopulmonary bypass and the usual cardiac surgical environment, although some groups have inserted the Thoratec VAD without cardiopulmonary bypass.[30] However, in some patients it is necessary to initiate cardiopulmonary bypass as a resuscitative measure. Patients who suffer sudden severe deterioration in the intensive care unit, emergency room, or cardiac catheterization laboratory can be placed on circulatory support systems using peripheral cannulation without the need for sternotomy. Systems have been developed for rapid placement of groin cannula,[31,32] and flows as high as 4 to 6 L/min can be obtained with these systems. If successful resuscitation is accomplished with a system using peripheral cannulation, plans should be made to change to the more sophisticated devices because it is doubtful that such peripheral systems can be maintained over the prolonged periods often required to obtain donor hearts. Unless a donor heart is readily available, these patients should have insertion of a more sophisticated device within 24 hours of resuscitation.

The position of the cannula and the pump should be carefully considered. If possible, devices should be positioned so that patients are able to be mobile. This is quite feasible with the external pulsatile devices such as the Thoratec and Symbion AVADs, the Novacor and Thermedics LVASs, and the Symbion TAH. Positioning of the Symbion TAH has been an important consideration in candidates who are being bridged to cardiac transplantation.[17] Since the development of the Jarvik-7-70, insertion has been greatly facilitated, especially in smaller men and women.

In selecting a device to support a patient before cardiac transplantation, it is advantageous to choose the system that requires minimal anticoagulation. The simpler systems such as ECMO and centrifugal pumps require continuous heparinization. With some of the more sophisticated systems, however, heparinization is less critical as long as the flow is maintained above 3 L/min. However, patients with the Novacor, Thoratec, Thermedics, Symbion TAH, and Symbion AVAD devices have almost all received some type of anticoagulation. The current regimen usually consists of treatment with continuous intravenous heparin as soon as the initial bleeding has stopped after implantation of the device (usually within 24 hr), in order to keep the partial thromboplastin time at 1.5 times control. For perfusions of longer durations, it is possible to change to warfarin and dipyridamole or aspirin. However, uniform anticoagulation protocols have not been defined for any of the devices mentioned in this chapter. Some investigators have been hesitant to use aspirin because of the danger of bleeding at the time of transplantation. Thromboembolic complications have been reported, regardless of the device used. At present, none of the systems mentioned can be relied on to function without the threat of thromboembolism, even if anticoagulation is employed. However, the incidence of death or severe stroke seems to be decreasing with better anticoagulation regimens. Bleeding is a common complication, occurring in more than 50% of our patients receiving assist devices.[33] We have used several techniques to control bleeding, including meticulous surgical technique, reversal of heparin used for cardiopulmonary bypass, generous applications of Surgicel, fibrin glue, and topical thrombin. However, the bleeding is often diffuse and sometimes related to coagulopathy. This necessitates the administration of large quantities of fresh frozen plasma and platelets. Pulsatile devices create stress at the suture lines used to place the pump outflow grafts to the aorta or pulmonary artery. Reinforcement with pledgeted mattress sutures often is necessary to control bleeding. We now attempt to close the sternum in all patients being bridged to transplantation. This has the advantage of limiting bleeding from the sternal edges and allowing for mobilization during the period before transplantation. Sometimes there is hemodynamic deterioration as a result of wiring the sternum, in which case the sternal wires have to be removed with only the subcutaneous tissue and skin closed.

Infection is another area of great concern for patients who are being bridged to cardiac transplantation. Since these patients will be immuno-suppressed after transplantation, the presence of a pretransplant infection may often exclude them as reasonable transplant candidates. Many patients had externalized pumps that necessitated cannulae passing through the abdominal or chest wall. The incidence of cannulae infection in these patients has been relatively low. Some patients with LVAS systems acquired infections at the site where the power cable exits the skin, but these local infections usually were treated effectively with local care and topical antibiotics. Infection of the abdominal pump pocket in these patients has also been documented[34]; however, there have been too few implantable devices used to determine the frequency of this complication. Infectious complications in patients receiving externalized systems as well as implantable LVAS systems seemed to be related more to time than to position of the pump and/or cannulae. A recent report from the University of Pittsburgh documented a high instance of mediastinal infections in patients who were bridged to transplantation with a Jarvik-7 TAH.[35] In this study, the infectious complications were not related to time; however, it was believed that positioning of the TAH itself within a "dead space" in the mediastinum placed the patient at a high risk for infection. Device-related infectious complications are rare after transplantation in patients receiving implantable or external VADs. Unfortunately, this did not appear to be true for patients who received TAHs.

Multiple organ failure, particularly renal failure, has been another obstacle to survival in patients undergoing mechanical circulatory support.[36] Renal or cerebral damage often occurs before placement of the assist device. In these patients, the cerebral and renal damage is usually not reversed by re-establishing adequate perfusion. Although there are patients who have survived renal dialysis after transplantation,[2] the survival rate in this group can be expected to be low.

The initial goal of circulatory support is to establish normal cardiac output and blood pressure as quickly as possible to avoid or reverse the ischemic injury to vital organs. Blood flow of at least 2 L/m^2 per min is imperative for survival. The actual drive parameters vary depending on which device is used. It has never been proven that synchronizing techniques facilitate ventricular recovery or improve device performance. However, the patients discussed in this chapter will not usually have myocardial recovery and, therefore, weaning techniques and synchronization are not important. Initially, the use of BVADs was feared to present problems of synchronization of the left and right pumps, but this has not been an important clinical problem. Regardless of which drive parameters are employed, synchronization of the pumps is not necessary. Obviously, a TAH does not have the problem of working in synchrony with the natural heart because the ventricles have been removed.

The placement of mechanical devices for temporary support can provide a screening period during which poor risk candidates with previously ill-defined prohibitive problems can be clearly identified. These patients may be rejected as cardiac transplant recipients, thus allowing for better allocation of donor organs. Additionally, the use of mechanical devices may provide a period during which the patient's overall condition can be improved by vigorous diuresis to reduce edema, increasing nutrition and muscle strength, and allowing time for resolution of major organ ischemia induced by prior low cardiac output can all be accomplished during support. The number of bridge-to-transplant patients is increasing yearly, as is the amount of time needed to locate a donor heart. For this reason, it is especially important that the patients become ambulatory, thus decreasing problems associated with being bedridden, such as atelectasis and muscle wasting.

At the time of transplantation, the patient is transported to the operating room. Cardiopulmonary bypass is initiated through either the groin or chest. All prosthetic graft material should be removed from the great vessels to prevent a source for infection. After removal of the devices, the tracts created by cannulae or drivelines may be packed open. In our experience, these wounds have not healed as quickly in the immunosuppressed patients as in our other patients, but they have all healed without infection or residual problems after transplantation.

Conclusions

A limited number of bridge-to-transplant procedures will be performed per year. Two factors limit the use of assist devices in this patient population: one is the increasing competition for a limited number of donor hearts and the other is the development of mechanical devices for long-term use. Electrical implantable LVASs may be available for clinical trials as early as next year. Once these devices become available, the need for mechanical support before cardiac transplantation will become less important. The supply of donor hearts could increase over the next several years; however, it is doubtful if more than 200 to 300 bridge-to-transplant procedures will ever be performed annually. Fifteen thousand patients per year require heart replacement. With only 1400 heart transplants performed in the United States in 1988, it can be assumed that, in the future, patients with permanent mechanical devices will greatly outnumber those with cardiac transplants.

References

1. Evans RW, Mannion DL, Garrison LP Jr, Maier AM. Donor availability as the primary determinant of the future of heart transplantation. *JAMA*. 1986;255:1892–1898.

2. Farrar DJ, Hill JD, Gray LA Jr, et al. Heterotopic prosthetic ventricles as a bridge to cardiac transplantation. *N Engl J Med.* 1988;318(6):333–340.
3. Joyce LD, Johnson KE, Pierce WS, et al. Summary of the world experience with clinical use of total artificial heart as heart support devices. *J Heart Transplant.* 1986;5:229–235.
4. Starnes VA, Oyer PE, Portner PM, et al. Isolated left ventricular assist as bridge to transplantation. *J Thorac Cardiovasc Surg.* 1988;96:62–71.
5. Bolman RM, Spray TL, Cox JL, et al. Heart transplantation in patients requiring preoperative mechanical support. *J Heart Transplant.* 1987;6:273–280.
6. Cooley DA, Liotta D, Hallman GL, Bloodwell RD, Leachman RD, Milam JD. Orthotopic cardiac prosthesis for two-staged cardiac replacement. *Am J Cardiol.* 1969;24:723–730.
7. Frazier OH, Painvin GA, Urrutia CO, Igo SR, Cooley DA. Mechanical circulatory support: clinical experience at the Texas Heart Institute. *J Heart Transplant.* 1983;2:299–306.
8. Reemstma K, Krusin R, Edie R, Bregman D, Dobelle W, Hardy M. Cardiac transplantation in patients requiring mechanical circulatory support. *N Engl J Med.* 1978;298:670–671.
9. Pennington DG, Codd JE, Merjavy JP, et al. The expanded use of ventricular bypass systems for severe cardiac failure and as a bridge to cardiac transplantation. *J Heart Transplant.* 1984;3:170–175.
10. Hardesty RL, Griffith BP, Trento A, Thompson ME, Fesson PF, Bahnson HT. Mortally ill patients and excellent survival following cardiac transplantation. *Ann Thorac Surg.* 1986;41:126–129.
11. Pennington DG, Merjavy JP, Codd JE, et al. Extracorporeal membrane oxygenation for patients with cardiogenic shock. *Circulation.* 1984;70(suppl I):130–137.
12. Williams BA, Lough ME, Shinn JA. Left ventricular assist device as a bridge to heart transplantation: a case study. *J Heart Transplant.* 1987;6:23–28.
13. Hill JD, Farrar DJ, Hirshon JJ, Compton PG, Avery GJ, Brent BN. Use of a prosthetic ventricle as a bridge to transplantation for postinfarction cardiogenic shock. *N Engl J Med.* 1986;314:626–628.
14. Levinson MM, Smith RG, Cork R, et al. Three recent cases of the total artificial heart before transplantation. *J Heart Transplant.* 1986;5:215–228.
15. Ganzel BL, Gray LA, Slater AD, Mavroudis C. Surgical techniques for the implantation of heterotopic prosthetic ventricles. *Ann Thorac Surg.* 1989;47:113–120.
16. Kanter KR, McBride LR, Pennington DG, et al. Bridging to cardiac transplantation with pulsatile ventricular assist devices. *Ann Thorac Surg.* 1988;46:134–140.
17. Jarvik RK, DeVries WC, Semb KHB. Surgical positioning of the Jarvik-7 total artificial heart. *J Heart Transplant.* 1986;5(3):184–195.
18. Park SB, Liebler GA, Burkholder JA, et al. Mechanical support of the failing heart. *Ann Thorac Surg.* 1986;42:627–632.
19. Pennington DG, Samuels LD, Williams GA, et al. Experience with the Pierce-Donachy ventricular assist device in postcardiotomy patients with cardiogenic shock. *World J Surg.* 1985;9:37–46.
20. Rose DM, Laschinger J, Grossi E, Krieger KH, Cunningham JN, Spencer FC. Experimental and clinical results with a simplified left heart assist device for treatment of profound left ventricular dysfunction. *World J Surg.* 1985;9:11–17.

21. Pennington DG, Kanter KR, McBride LR, et al. Seven years' experience with the Pierce-Donachy ventricular assist device. *J Thorac Cardiovasc Surg.* 1988,96:901–911.
22. Pennington DG, McBride LR, Swartz MT, et al. The effect of perioperative myocardial infarction on survival of postcardiotomy patients supported with ventricular assist devices. *Circulation.* 1988;78:(suppl III)110–115.
23. Pennington DG, Merjavy JP, Swartz MT, et al. The importance of biventricular failure in patients with postoperative cardiogenic shock. *Ann Thorac Surg.* 1985;39:16–26.
24. Litwak RS, Koffsky RM, Jurado RA, Mitchell BA, King P. A decade of experience with a left heart assist device in patients undergoing open intracardiac operation. *World J Surg.* 1985;9:18–24.
25. Norman JC, Duncan JH, Frazier OH, et al. Intracorporeal (abdominal) left ventricular assist devices or partial artificial hearts. *Arch Surg.* 1981;116:1441–1445.
26. Bernhard WF, Berger RL, Stetz JP, et al. Temporary left ventricular bypass: factors affecting patient survival. *Circulation.* 1979;60(2)(suppl I):131–140.
27. Swartz MT, Pennington DG, Ruzevich S, et al. The incidence of isolated left ventricular failure in bridge to transplant patients. *Trans Am Soc Artif Intern Organs.* 1989;35:730–733.
28. Golding LR, Stewart RW, Sinkewich M, Smith W, Cosgrove DM. Nonpulsatile ventricular assist bridging to transplantation. *Trans Am Soc Artif Intern Organs.* 1988;34:476–479.
29. Joyce LD, Johnson K, Cabrol C, et al. Results of the first one hundred patients who received Jarvik total artificial hearts as a bridge to transplantation. *Circulation.* 1988;78(suppl II):581.
30. Brugger JP, Bonandi L, Meli M, et al. Swat team approach to ventricular assistance. *Ann Thorac Surg.* 1989;47:136–141.
31. Wampler RK, Moise JC, Frazier OH, et al. "In vivo" evaluation of a peripheral vascular access axial flow blood pump. *Trans Am Soc Intern Organs.* 1988;34:450–454.
32. Kanter KR, Pennington DG, Vandermael M, et al. Emergency resuscitation with extracorporeal membrane oxygenation for failed angioplasty. *J Am Coll Cardiol.* 1988;11:149. Abstract.
33. Swartz MT, Pennington DG, McBride LR, et al. Temporary mechanical circulatory support: clinical experience with 148 patients. In: Unger F, ed. *Assisted Circulation 2.* Berlin-Heidelberg: Springer-Verlag; 1989:132–151.
34. Reedy JE, Ruzevich SA, Swartz MT, Termuhlen DF, Pennington DG. Nursing care of a patient requiring prolonged mechanical circulatory support. *Prog Cardiovasc Nurs.* 1989;4:1–9.
35. Griffith BP, Kormos RL, Hardesty RL, et al. The artificial heart: infection-related morbidity and its effect on transplantation. *Ann Thorac Surg.* 1988;45:409–414.
36. Kanter KR, Swartz MT, Pennington DG, et al. Renal failure in patients with ventricular assist devices. *Trans Am Soc Artif Intern Organs.* 1987;33:426–428.

5
Recipient Selection for Cardiac Transplantation

GEORGE A. PANTELY

The primary goal of heart transplantation is to prolong life in people with a severe, irreversible reduction in cardiac function. A secondary aspect of this goal is to restore the quality of life to or near normal. Criteria for selecting individuals to undergo heart transplantation to achieve these goals have been recommended.[1] However, each program develops a philosophy about selecting individuals for heart transplantation.[2] Some prefer to follow the criteria relatively unchanged from that developed at Stanford in the 1970s,[3,4] whereas others have a philosophy of challenging accepted criteria and making heart transplantation available to a broader spectrum of individuals.[5] This has led to substantial modification of the patient selection criteria in recent years. However, all centers are faced with the same major limitation in selecting individuals to undergo heart transplantation—the number of people who would benefit from a heart transplant far exceeds the supply of donor hearts available.[6] Centers try to maintain a reasonable balance between the number of patients accepted as heart transplant candidates and the number of donor hearts available to a center. Thus, despite a desire to make heart transplantation available to a broad spectrum of individuals, the limited number of donor hearts does require a selection process from the group of individuals who are potential candidates to undergo this procedure.

In discussing the selection of patients for heart transplantation, primary emphasis will be placed on identifying those individuals whose survival and quality of life will be improved substantially by the procedure. Second, other factors that are considered to help assure the greatest likelihood of a successful operation, recovery, and long-term survival will be discussed. It will be evident that it is in the consideration of these factors that the philosophy of a center and the limitations of donor supply lead to variability in selection criteria. Third, a suggested evaluation that a patient should undergo will also be outlined.

Establishing Criteria for Heart Transplant Recipients

Table 5.1 lists generally accepted criteria for selecting candidates for heart transplantation.

TABLE 5.1. Criteria for selecting candidates for heart transplantation.

I. Specific indications:
  A. Severe, irreversible reductions in heart function (EF[a] <20–25%) with disabling symptoms of heart failure (FC III-late or IV)
  B. Patients judged to have a substantial and imminent risk of cardiac death despite not fully meeting the criteria listed above
  C. Other reasonable medical and surgical options are not available
II. No other conditions that might limit the success of heart transplantation should be present. Factors to consider:
  A. Absence of pulmonary vascular disease. PVR should be <6–8 Wood units and pulmonary artery pressure <50–60 mmHg (concern: limited work capacity of the normal right ventricle)
  B. Age <55 years. In many centers, this has been extended to age <60 years with carefully selected patients >60 years considered (concern: diminished capacity to withstand the procedure or increased incidence of postoperative complications)
  C. Absence of active infection or potential sources of infection (concern: exacerbation with immunosuppression)
  D. Absence of significant renal (creatinine <2 mg/dl and creatinine clearance >50 ml/min) and hepatic (bilirubin, SGPT, SGOT <twice normal) function (concern: exacerbation resulting from procedure and immunosuppression)
  E. Absence of insulin-requiring diabetes. Many centers will consider insulin-requiring diabetics who are well controlled and who have no evidence of end-organ damage (concern: exacerbation by chronic corticosteroid therapy)
  F Absence of significant pulmonary disease—FEV_1[b]/FVC[c] >50% and FEV^1 >50% of predicted (concern: increased perioperative pulmonary complications and infections)
  G. Absence of psychosocial instability and inadequate supportive social situation (concern: if history of behavior problems, addictions, or illness, patient will not comply with life-long medical regimen and required daily medications with life-threatening complications in event of noncompliance)
  H. Absence of significant crossmatch incompatibility between donor and recipient (concern: greater likelihood of uncontrollable rejection)
  I. Lack of other co-existing medical problems that might limit life expectancy or compromise the chance of a successful heart transplantation. Things to evaluate (but not necessarily exclude) patients for are:
    1. Symptomatic or severe asymptomatic peripheral or cerebral vascular disease
    2. Addictive diseases such as alcoholism and illicit drug use
    3. Previous malignancy (concern: increased risk of recurrence or new malignancy)
    4. Amyloidosis (concern: recurrence in transplanted heart)
    5. HIV-antibody positive (concern: activation of AIDS)
    6. Jehovah's Witness (concern: unable to use blood or blood products)

[a]EF = ejection fraction.
[b]FEV_1 = forced expiratory volume in 1 second.
[c]FVC = forced vital capacity.

TABLE 5.2. Survival after heart transplantation.

	Survival (%)		
	ISHT[a]		
Years after transplant	All patients	Triple RX	CHTS[b]
1	78	87	78
3	75	84	68
5	73	83	—

[a]ISHT = International Society for Heart Transplantation Registry. Approximate survival extracted from Fig. 9 in ref. 7. All patients = all patients reported to the registry. Triple RX = subgroup of more recently transplanted patients who have been treated with cyclosporine, azathioprine, and prednisone.
[b]CHTS = Collaborative Heart Transplant Study Registry. Approximate survival extracted from the figure in ref. 8. Data up to 5 years posttransplant are not available.

Severe, Irreversible Reductions in Heart Function with Disabling Symptoms of Heart Failure

Cardiac transplantation is indicated in patients with end-stage heart disease whose survival with optimal standard therapy is judged to be severely limited compared to survival after heart transplantation and when no other reasonable medical or surgical options are available.

Data for survival after heart transplantation have been collected by two major registries—the International Society for Heart Transplantation[7] started in 1983 and the Collaborative Heart Transplant Study,[8] which was initiated in the spring of 1985. Data from many centers are included in both registries, although some centers report to only one registry. The survival data from each registry are reasonably similar, as shown in Table 5.2.

Patients with end-stage heart disease whose survival is estimated to be substantially worse than shown in Table 5.2 should be considered for heart transplantation. "Substantially worse" survival is generally defined as an estimated 50% or less survival after 1 year. The estimated life expectancy in some patients with end-stage heart disease may be straightforward. Those in hospital requiring mechanical circulatory support, inotropic agents, and antiarrhythmic agents to prevent recurrent ventricular tachycardia/fibrillation are unlikely to survive for an extended period without heart transplant. Predicting 1-year survival in most individuals with more stable, but yet end-stage heart disease, however, is uncertain at best. In general, patients with an ejection fraction of 20% to 25% or less and who are New York Heart Association (NYHA) functional Class III (late) or IV fit the category of having "substantially worse" survival.[9,10] In general, these individuals cannot perform the simple activities of daily living without fatigue or dyspnea. Other factors determined by multivariant analysis that indicate a poor prognosis are the presence of left ventricular conduction delay on the electrocardiogram (ECG), marked elevation of pulmonary capillary wedge (PCW) pressure (>25–30 mmHg), complex ventricular arrhythmias, and elevated right atrial pressure (>10 mmHg).[9,11]

Interestingly, some individuals with ejection fractions in this range may be functional Class II or III (early). These people are usually maintained on medical therapy until a deterioration of functional class has occurred. However, the 1-year survival of these people who are considered "too well" for heart transplantation may also be substantially reduced.[12] Thus, the value of using functional class (FC) to determine prognosis and the timing of heart transplantation is not ideal. At present, patients with heart failure in FC II or III (early) are not usually considered for transplant. This is reasonable until better methods are available to risk-stratify patients with end-stage heart disease and preserved FC, the mortality for heart transplant and complications of immunosuppression are further reduced, and the supply-to-demand ratio of available donor hearts improves.

Individuals with severe left ventricular dysfunction not related to coronary artery disease and a brief duration of symptoms (weeks to several months) should have the decision for heart transplantation delayed if possible. Left ventricular function has been reported to improve significantly in about 20% of such individuals, delaying or eliminating the need for heart transplantation.[13,14]

Certain individuals with limited symptoms of heart failure and only moderate reductions in left ventricular function may be considered for heart transplant if the risk for cardiac death is judged to be substantial and imminent. Such cases are fortunately infrequent. This situation might arise in a patient with severe, life-threatening episodes of myocardial ischemia (pulmonary edema, hypotension, and ventricular arrhythmias) that persist despite therapy and that cannot be relieved or improved by cardiac surgery.

Other Factors That Might Limit the Success of Heart Transplantation

Once it has been established that the cardiac disease is severe enough to warrant heart transplantation, it is important to exclude and/or correct other noncardiac factors that might limit the success of the heart transplantation and the opportunity for long-term survival.

Pulmonary Vascular Resistance

PVR (Wood units) is defined as mean pulmonary artery pressure (mmHg) minus mean PCW pressure (mmHg) divided by cardiac output (L/min).

Normal pulmonary vascular resistance (PVR) is <2.5 Wood units.

These arbitrary resistance units may be converted to absolute resistance units expressed in dynes-sec-cm^{-5} by multiplying Wood units by 80. The resting PVR and pulmonary artery pressure are often elevated in patients with severe congestive heart failure because of hypoxia or secondary to markedly elevated left ventricular filling pressures. In these situations, having the patient breathe oxygen-enriched air or administering a vasodilator or inotropic agent may lower left ventricular end-diastolic pressure and pulmonary pressure, leading to an increase in cardiac output.[15] The resultant fall in PVR indicates that the elevated PVR was secondary to the congestive heart failure and not a fixed increase in PVR.

A PVR elevated to or above 6 to 8 Wood units (480–640 dynes-sec-cm^{-5}) and/or a pulmonary artery (PA) systolic pressure >50 to 60 mmHg despite oxygen or medication are strong contraindications to orthotonic heart transplantation.[16,17] Acute right ventricular dilation and failure of the donor heart leading to death is likely to occur because the right ventricle cannot acutely generate the high pressures necessary to pump blood through the pulmonary vascular bed. The extent of the elevated PVR and mortality posttransplant may vary continuously rather than showing a steep increase in mortality at a specific PVR of 6 to 8 Wood units.[18] This does not lend support to establishing precise levels of PVR and PA systolic pressures for transplant candidates, but rather emphasizes the need to recognize that any elevation of PVR and PA systolic pressures may add some risk to the procedure.

Several options have been suggested to enable heart transplantation in patients with elevated PVR. These include: (1) using a larger donor heart, (2) using a donor heart "prepared" to handle a high PVR (e.g., the rare situation of obtaining a heart from an individual undergoing heart-lung transplant where the right ventricle was exposed to high PVR, but the heart is otherwise normal), (3) performing heart-lung transplantation, and (4) performing a heterotopic heart transplant. Insufficient data are available to support the usefulness of these options, but the first is used most commonly.

Age

An upper age limit of 50 years initially was established for heart transplantation. This was based on Stanford's early experience showing that patients older than 50 years had a 1-year survival of 50% and a 5-year survival of 23%. This contrasted with a 70% 1-year and a 50% 5-year survival in younger patients.[17] The age criteria have been extended gradually so that now patients between 50 and 60 years old are routinely considered for transplant and selected patients older than 60 years are considered in many centers. Data from the International Society for Heart Transplantation Registry[7] indicate that approximately 25% of heart transplants performed in 1988 were in patients older than 55 years. Recent reports have indicated no increased mortality or morbidity in patients older than 55 years,[7,19-21] although the number of patients involved is small and the duration of follow-up is short.

The debate about suitable age for heart transplantation is multifaceted. One argument is that if the number of available donor hearts exceeds the number of candidates under 55 years of age, these hearts should not be wasted, but used in selected older patients. In addition, since available results do not show increased problems in the elderly, no medical reason exists to deny transplantation. This must be balanced against worsening the existing problem of an insufficient number of donor hearts and the total cost of heart transplantation compared to standard management of end-stage heart disease. Thus, the issue of age is unresolved at present and previously established limits are being challenged. Current practice in most centers is to consider patients between 50 and 60 years of age routinely and selectively consider patients older than 60 years for heart transplantation. This is reasonable until data are available to suggest that other approaches are indicated.

Absence of Active Infection and Potential Sources of Infection

Patients should be free of active infection at the time of transplantation. Those individuals with evidence of an untreated, indolent infection (a positive tuberculin skin test) should have appropriate treatment. Any potential source of infection should be eliminated before surgery. This most commonly includes removal or repair of teeth. Another example is a recent pulmonary emboli with lung infarction. Such patients may develop a lung infection and abscess with immunosuppression postoperatively.[22] Surgery should be delayed until the necrotic tissue is cleared, which may take 6 to 8 weeks.

Normal Renal and Hepatic Function or Reversible Dysfunction

Patients should have normal or near normal renal (creatinine <2 mg/dl and creatinine clearance >50 ml/min) and hepatic (bilirubin, serum glutamic pyruvic transaminase, serum glutamic oxaloacetic transaminase less than twice normal) function before heart transplantation. Function of these organs, especially the kidneys, is often impaired by immunosuppression therapy (especially cyclosporine A) after transplantation. Preexisting dysfunction is usually accentuated by the immunosuppression therapy. If renal and hepatic function are not normal, the cause should be sought and corrected if possible. Severe congestive heart failure often causes mild to moderate abnormalities in laboratory values looking at the function of these two organs.[23,24] The degree of the abnormalities may fluctuate with changes in cardiac status. These abnormalities are usually reversible after heart transplantation. Congestive heart failure is the likely cause if only mild to moderate chemical abnormalities are present and the patient has no evidence of end-organ disease on history, physical examination, or noninvasive testing.

Insulin-Requiring Diabetes

The concern in performing heart transplantation in this group has been the increased risk of infection and the difficulty in controlling the diabetes with prednisone immunosuppression. Diabetes is also associated with a higher incidence of other vascular disease and renal disease. The result after renal transplantation in diabetic patients has been acceptable. Young diabetic patients without retinopathy, neuropathy, or nephropathy are now considered for heart transplantation at many centers. Short-term results show no major problems, except for a higher incidence of rejection in the first months posttransplant that is likely related to attempts to withdraw or use minimal prednisone.[25] The long-term prognosis in these patients has not been established. Based on current information, it is reasonable to consider heart transplantation in select patients with diabetes and without evidence of end-organ damage.

Chronic, Severe Pulmonary Disease

Patients become less suitable candidates for transplantation as the degree of pulmonary dysfunction increases. Severe chronic bronchitis or chronic obstructive pulmonary disease may cause problems in the perioperative period and may increase the risk of pulmonary infection during immunosuppression therapy. The evaluation of pulmonary function is complicated because it is adversely compromised by severe congestive heart failure.[26] General guidelines are that individuals with severe airway obstruction forced expiratory volume in 1 sec to forced vital capacity (FEV^1/FVC) ratio of <45–50% of predicted) or severe restrictive disease (FEV <50% of predicted) despite optimal medical therapy are poor candidates.

Psychosocial Stability and Adequate Supportive Social Situation

It is difficult to establish firm criteria in these areas. The goal is to be confident that the individual is capable of taking care of his needs, will reliably take his medications, and will comply with the biopsy, laboratory tests, and out-patient appointments that are a part of life after a heart transplant. Thorough evaluations of the individual and the extended family by a psychiatrist and social worker are helpful in identifying any problems. Efforts should be made to correct potentially life-threatening problems before excluding a patient from transplantation. If the patient is medically stable, this might involve a period of observation to see if the individual will comply with specific requests or treatment schedules and refrain from addictive behavior.

Crossmatch Incompatibility Between Recipient and Donor

The presence of high levels of preformed antibodies in the recipient's serum to a random panel of lymphocytes may indicate a higher likelihood for acute rejection or greater difficulty in controlling chronic rejection.[27] This occurs when the patient's preformed antibodies reacted strongly to the donor lymphocytes in vitro. This problem may be overcome by performing a prospective crossmatch to assure that such a patient would receive a heart only from a donor with whom the patient has a negative or weakly positive crossmatch. The mechanics of performing a prospective crossmatch make this a difficult test to perform except when the potential donor is within a short distance of the transplant center. Areas of investigation include methods to remove preformed antibodies by a variety of plasmaphoresis techniques that hopefully would ultimately enable highly sensitized individuals to undergo transplantation and potentially eliminate the need for prospective crossmatching.

Co-existing Medical Problems That May Limit Life Expectancy or Compromise the Chance of a Successful Heart Transplant

A long list of medical problems can be constructed that may preclude or significantly compromise the chance of a successful heart transplantation. However, little definitive information is available to aid in decisionmaking, and substantial variability exists between centers in the importance placed on any given factor. A few specific issues will be discussed.

Symptomatic or Severe Asymptomatic Peripheral or Cerebral Vascular Disease

The concerns are that the vascular disease may progress more rapidly, that the patients will have a greater risk for strokes, and that they will require additional surgical procedures for the vascular disease that will be associated with increased morbidity and perhaps mortality.

Addictive Diseases

Active addictive diseases such as alcoholism and illicit, drug use should exclude an individual. These habits may be the cause of the heart damage and need to be terminated to prevent potential damage to the transplanted heart. Lack of compliance in taking medications will be life-threatening in these individuals. A past history of addictive behavior (6 months to 1 year previously) is not necessarily exclusive, but objective evidence that the individual is free of his addictions should be sought.

Previous Malignancy

People who have been "cured" of a malignancy are referred for heart transplantation after developing a cardiomyopathy secondary to radiation therapy or chemotherapeutic drugs. The concern is that the immunosuppression therapy after transplantation may reactivate the malignancy or that these people may be at increased risk for developing a second malignancy. Heart transplantation has been performed in a small number of selected patients who were felt to be free of any recurrence for at least 1 year[28]; however, long-term follow-up will be required to establish the risk in these individuals for recurrence or new malignancies to develop.

Amyloidosis

The initial experience with transplantation in individuals with amyloidosis was accidental with the diagnosis being made retrospectively during examination of the explanted heart. More recently, individuals known to have amyloidosis have been transplanted.[29] None of these individuals had other end-organ dysfunction despite evidence of amyloid in other organs. One individual has recurrent cardiac amyloidosis detectable only by electron microscopy.[30] The intermediate-term results in these individuals have been good; long-term results have not been established.

Human Immunodeficiency Virus Antibody-Positive Individuals

Candidates for heart transplantation at our center undergo human immunodeficiency virus (HIV) testing to screen for antibody-positive individuals. To date we have not been confronted with making the decision whether to transplant an individual who is antibody-positive without any evidence of the disease. If such cases exist, none have been reported in the literature. The concerns are that the virus may cause damage to the transplanted heart or that immunosuppression may cause a more rapid onset of the disease. No information is available to help make this decision. As most of the "contraindications" to heart transplant have been challenged, one anticipates that such individuals may be transplanted in the future.

Jehovah's Witness

Transplant programs may be reluctant to perform heart transplantation in people of the Jehovah's Witness faith because it must be done without the use of supplemental blood or blood products. The goal to prolong life could thus be thwarted by the lack of a blood transfusion, a commonplace and simple life-saving procedure. We have performed successful heart transplantation in a carefully selected Jehovah's Witness who did not have prior open heart surgery. Two other cases have been reported.[31,32] Previous open heart surgery may preclude performing heart transplantation without using blood products.

Recipient Evaluation

The recipient evaluation is designed to (1) determine the etiology of the cardiac disease, (2) quantify functional class, cardiac function, and PVR, and (3) exclude active diseases or organ dysfunction that preclude transplantation or should delay transplantation until the problem is resolved.

Determine the Etiology of the Cardiac Disease

Coronary angiography and endomyocardial biopsy may be done to establish the etiology of the cardiac dysfunction and to be sure that alternative procedures are not indicated that could improve cardiac function. This includes mainly bypass graft surgery or angioplasty for severe ischemia that results in left ventricular dysfunction that is reversible when ischemia is relieved. Myocarditis and other rare diseases (cardiac sarcoidosis and giant cell myocarditis), which are diagnosed by endomyocardial biopsy, are potentially treatable with improvement in ventricular function. The clinical merit of an endomyocardial biopsy in defining the etiology of congestive heart failure is limited and probably need only be done in patients suspected of having acute myocarditis.[33] Even in this group, only 10% of individuals will have myocarditis found on the biopsy samples. Coronary angiography and endomyocardial biopsy, or other attempts to define the etiology of heart failure, may be unnecessary in individuals with a long, established history of a cardiomyopathy or clear-cut evidence of coronary artery disease without evidence of ongoing ischemia as the cause of cardiac dysfunction and whose ejection fraction is less than 20% on noninvasive studies. It is unlikely that cardiac function can be improved by any intervention; the risks of these tests may exceed any anticipated benefit.

Establish Cardiac Function and Pulmonary Vascular Resistance

Ventricular function must be quantitated. This can be achieved by left ventricular angiography, radionuclide ventriculography (perhaps the preferred method), or echocardiography. The individual's functional class can usually be obtained by history or by watching the patient walk or trying to climb stairs. A modified exercise test (modified Bruce or Naughton) can be used to clarify and quantify functional class.

A right heart catheterization with measurement of pressures and thermodilution cardiac output should be performed in all patients to determine hemodynamic status and PVR. This is ideally done when the individual is on optimal therapy. If the PVR is elevated above normal (>3 Wood units), nitroprusside can be infused according to the protocol shown in Table 5.3 while blood pressure and heart rate are monitored. This is continued until the PVR falls to <3 Wood units or hypotension intervenes, preventing further attempts to lower PVR. A fall in the PVR with nitroprusside is used to confirm that the elevated PVR is secondary to high left-sided filling pressure and not fixed pulmonary vascular disease.

Exclude Active Illness or Significant Organ Dysfunction

The physician must exclude active illness or significant organ dysfunction by a thorough physical examination, extensive laboratory testing, and in-

TABLE 5.3. Protocol for determining the pulmonary vascular resistance and pulmonary artery pressure during nitroprusside infusion.

1. Perform a right heart catheterization using a balloon-tipped thermodilution cardiac output catheter
2. Obtain baseline hemodynamic measurements, cardiac output, and calculate the PVR
3. If the PVR is >3 Wood units or PA systolic pressure is >50–60 mmHg, begin continuous intravenous infusion of nitroprusside at 0.5 μg/kg/min. Increase the infusion rate by 0.5 μg/kg/min every 3–5 min based on systemic blood pressure obtained by a cuff and/or patient symptoms
4. Repeat the hemodynamic and cardiac output measurements and calculate the PVR. The nitroprusside infusion can be increased until the PVR falls to <3 Wood units or hypotension intervenes, preventing further attempts to lower the PVR

vestigation of any significant or unexpected abnormalities. Table 5.4 provides a list for the evaluation of patients at the Oregon Health Sciences University. This table is provided only as an example and is expanded or contracted as indicated for a given individual. The evaluation is modified if the patient is critically ill and unable to undergo specific tests.

When the evaluation is complete, the case is presented to the group responsible for reviewing the data and recommending individuals for heart transplantation. This group usually includes cardiologists, cardiac surgeons, transplant physicians, psychiatrist, and social worker. Some centers include lay people and physicians not directly involved in transplantation in their review group. This review enables identification of potential problems and the formation of plans to deal with problems.

Conclusions

The primary goal of heart transplantation is to prolong survival and improve the quality of life in individuals with a severe, uncorrectable reduction in heart function. The purpose of the evaluation process outlined in this chapter is not only to identify patients most likely to benefit from the procedure, but who also will have the greatest likelihood of a successful operation, recovery, and long-term survival.

The criteria are not designed to be exclusionary, but rather to make heart transplantation as safe and successful as possible for the patient. No firm policies have been established; rather, each center has been allowed to develop its own philosophy toward heart transplantation and to modify accepted criteria for candidate selection. The "conservative" criteria to select candidates for heart transplantation are being challenged and are now more "liberal" in an attempt to include more patients for whom the procedure has a reasonable chance of success. This has been done without a significant increase in short-term mortality or morbidity. However, expansion of the criteria is not without its problems. The major limitation to heart transplantation is still that the number of potential can-

TABLE 5.4. Heart transplantation evaluation.

I. Complete history and physical examination
II. Special diagnostic studies
    A. Coronary angiography (if indicated)
    B. Endomyocardial biopsy (if indicated)
    C. Quantitative left ventricular ejection fraction by radionuclide ventriculography (echocardiography or contrast ventriculography also options)
    D. Quantitation of PVR and PA systolic pressure with nitroprusside infusion if PVR >3 Wood units and PA systolic pressure >50–60 mmHg
    E. Echocardiogram
    F. Ambulatory ECG monitoring (if indicated)
III. Routine diagnostic studies
    A. Chest x-ray
    B. Electrocardiogram
    C. Pulmonary function tests with arterial blood gas and bronchodilators
    D. Stool guaiac times three
IV. Laboratory studies
    A. Complete blood count
    B. Fasting multichemical screening test
    C. Prothrombin time and partial thromboplastin time
    D. Ivy bleeding time
    E. Hepatitis screening tests
    F. Cholesterol and triglyceride levels
    G. Thyroid function panel
    H. Serum protein electrophoresis
    I. Antinuclear antibody and rheumatoid factor
    J. Blood type and screen
    K. Special immunologic studies for crossmatch incompatibility (panel of reactive antibodies)
    L. Rapid plasma reagin and toxoplasmosis titer
    M. Cytomegalic viral and Epstein-Barr titer
    N. Histoplasmosis titer (if resided in Midwest) and coccidiomycosis titer (if resided in Southwest)
    O. Pregnancy test (if applicable)
    P. Urine analysis
    Q. 24-hr urine collection for creatine clearance and protein
    R. PPD and 2 control skin tests; read results in 48 and 72 hr
V. Consultations
    A. Psychiatric evaluation
    B. Social worker evaluation
    C. Dental examination
    D. Financial counselor

didates far exceeds the number of donor hearts available. Expanding the criteria to make heart transplantation available to more patients has only aggravated that problem. It has also extended the waiting period and may result in more people dying while awaiting heart transplantation. The risks of expanding the criteria may ultimately be a reduced success rate. The final judgment about modification of the criteria awaits longer follow-up.

References

1. Health Care Financing Administration, Medical Program. Solicitation of hospitals and medical centers to participate in a study of heart transplant. *Fed Reg.* 1981;46:70–72.
2. Evans RW, Maier AM. Outcome of patients referred for cardiac transplantation. *J Am Coll Cardiol.* 1986;8:1312–1317.
3. Baumgartner WA, Reitz BA, Oyer PE, et al. Cardiac transplantation. *Curr Probl Surg.* 1979;16:2–61.
4. Copeland JG, Stinson EB. Human heart transplantation. *Curr Probl Cardiol.* 1979;4:1–51.
5. Copeland JG. Cardiac transplantation. *Curr Probl Cardiol.* 1988;13:157–224.
6. Evans RW, Manninen DL, Garrison LP, et al. Donor availability as the primary determinant of the future of heart transplantation. *JAMA.* 1986;255:1892–1898.
7. Fragomeni LS, Kaye MP. The registry of the International Society for Heart Transplantation. Fifth Official Report—1988. *J Heart Transplant.* 1988;7:249–253.
8. Opelz G. Collaborative heart transplant study. *Newsletter,* Feb. 14, 1989, no. 1.
9. Wilson JR, Schwartz JS, Sutton MSJ, et al. Prognosis in severe heart failure: relation to hemodynamic measurements and ventricular ectopic activity. *J Am Coll Cardiol.* 1983;2:403–410.
10. Franciosa JA, Wilen M, Ziesche S, et al. Survival in man with severe chronic left ventricular failure due to either coronary heart disease or idiopathic dilated cardiomyopathy. *Am J Cardiol.* 1983;51:831–836.
11. Unverferth DV, Magorien RD, Moeschberger ML, et al. Factors influencing the one-year mortality of dilated cardiomyopathy. *Am J Cardiol.* 1984;54:147–152.
12. Stevenson LW, Fowler MB, Schroeder JS, et al. Unexpected poor survival with dilated cardiomyopathy when transplantation denied due to limited symptoms. *Am J Med.* 1987;83:871–876.
13. Sekiguchi M, Hiroe M, Take M, et al. Natural history of 20 patients with biopsy proven acute myocarditis. A 10 year follow-up. *Circulation* 1985;72(suppl III):III–119. Abstract.
14. Strain JE, Grose RM, Cho S, et al. Short-term natural history of untreated myocarditis. *Circulation* 1985;72(suppl III):III–110. Abstract.
15. Schroeder JS. Current status of cardiac transplantation. *JAMA.* 1979;241:2069–2071.
16. Griepp RB, Stinson EB, Dong E, et al. Determinants of operative risk in human heart transplant. *Am J Surg.* 1971;122:192–197.
17. Baumgartner WA, Reitz BA, Oyer PE, et al. Cardiac homotransplantation. *Curr Probl Surg.* 1979;16:1–61.
18. Kirklin JK, Naftel DC, Kirklin JW, et al. Pulmonary vascular resistance and the risk of transplantation. *J Heart Transplant.* 1988;7:331–336.
19. Miller LW, Vitale-Noedel N, Pennington DG, et al. Heart transplantation in patients over age 55. *J Heart Transplant.* 1988;7:254–257.
20. Olivari MT, Antolick A, Kaye MP, et al. Heart transplant in elderly patients. *J Heart Transplant.* 1988;7:258–264.
21. Carrier M, Emery RW, Riley JE, et al. Cardiac transplantation in patients over the age of 50 years. *J Am Coll Cardiol.* 1986;8:285–288.

22. Young JN, Yazbeck J, Esposito G, et al. The influence of acute pre-operative pulmonary infarction on the results of cardiac transplantation. *J Heart Transplant* 1985;4:600. Abstract.
23. Pastan SO, Braunwald E. Renal disorders and heart disease. In: Braunwald E, ed. *Heart Disease*. Philadelphia: WB Saunders Co; 1988:1828–1835.
24. Kubo SH, Walter BA, John DHA, et al. Liver function abnormalities in chronic heart failure. Influence of systemic hemodynamics. *Arch Intern Med*. 1987;147:1227–1230.
25. Rhenman MJ, Rhenman B, Icenogle T, et al. Diabetes and heart transplantation. *J Heart Transplant*. 1988;7:356–358.
26. Light RW, George RB. Serial pulmonary function in patients with acute heart failure. *Arch Intern Med*. 1983;143:429–433.
27. Rabin BS. Immunologic aspects of human cardiac transplantation. *Heart Transplant*. 1983;2:188–191.
28. Armitage JM, Griffith BP, Kormos RL, et al. Cardiac transplantation in patients with malignancy. *J Heart Transplant*. 1989;8:89. Abstract.
29. Hosenpud JD, Uretsky BF, O'Connell JB, et al. Cardiac transplantation for amyloidosis. Results of a multicenter survey. *J Heart Transplant*. 1989;8:99. Abstract.
30. Connor R, Hosenpud JD, Norman DJ, et al. Transplantation for cardiac amyloidosis. Successful 1 year outcome despite recurrence of the disease. *J Heart Transplant*. 1988;7:165–167.
31. Corno AF, Laks H, Stevenson LW, et al. Heart transplantation in a Jehovah's Witness. *J Heart Transplant*. 1986;5:175–177.
32. Lammermeier DE, Duncan JM, Kuykendall RC, et al. Cardiac transplantation in a Jehovah's Witness. *Texas Heart Inst J*. 1988;15:189–192.
33. Mason JW, O'Connell JB. Clinical merit of endomyocardial biopsy. *Circulation*. 1989;79:971–979.

6
Donor Selection and Management for Cardiac Transplantation

JEFFREY SWANSON AND ADNAN COBANOGLU

With increasing experience and the advent of standardized protocols for the management of patients undergoing heart transplantation, the results obtained with this procedure have been gratifying and this mode of treatment has become widespread. In 1988, there were nearly 2500 heart transplants registered by the International Society for Heart Transplantation.[1] This represents an approximate eight-fold increase over the number recorded only 5 years earlier in 1983. The inevitable result of this burgeoning activity is to put pressure on the availability of suitable donor organs. In this context, the organ donor must be regarded as a precious natural resource that must be identified and preserved. The passage of the Uniform Anatomical Gift Act in 1968[2] and its acceptance by most states over the past two decades, in addition to the growing public awareness and acceptance of organ donation, has brought about an increase in the number of available organs. Most transplant centers have tried to further this increase by loosening acceptance criteria, thus making additional organs available. The evaluation of these potential donors in terms of their appropriateness for heart transplantation becomes a critical judgment in assuring a successful recipient outcome and avoiding organ waste. The medical management of these donors is critical in maintaining stable organ perfusion and metabolic homeostasis up to the time the organ is actually removed.

Donor Identification

Early identification of the organ donor is important in minimizing the period of time until actual procurement. Typically, the organ donor will present through the emergency room as a victim of blunt or penetrating head injury, subarachnoid hemorrhage or anoxic brain damage related to strangulation, drowning, or poisoning. They require endotracheal intubation and mechanical ventilation and frequently require volume resuscitation for blood loss from associated injuries or from loss of vasomotor tone. After initial emergency resuscitation, these patients are found in the intensive care unit environment where brain death is suspected.

TABLE 6.1. Clinical and laboratory findings in brain death.

Absence of cortical function
Spontaneous movement (nonreflexive)
Response to external stimuli
Response to pain
Absence of brain stem function
Spontaneous respiration
Pupillary response
Corneal reflex
Occulocephalic response (doll's eyes)
Vestibulooccular response (caloric)
Absence of electrocerebral activity (EEG)
Absence of cerebral blood flow

Medical Criteria for Brain Death

Table 6.1 lists the clinical and laboratory findings in brain death. The confirmation of brain death is a pivotal determination and can be suspected in a patient who is comatose and totally unresponsive to all stimuli.[3,4] Deep pain, produced by pressure on the supraorbital nerve, the tip of the mastoid process, or by squeezing the pectoralis major muscle, should produce no movement or pupillary dilatation. The pupils should show no response to strong light. Spontaneous respirations are absent, as are other brain stem reflexes.[5] Corneal reflexes, oculocephalic (doll's eye) response, and gag and cough reflexes are all absent, and there is no vestibuloocular (caloric) response.[5] Nevertheless, spinal reflexes can persist in patients who are brain dead.[6] The lack of respiratory effort can be confirmed by an "apnea test,"[7] but this examination is imprecise if only a limited time of observation is used. In fact, the threshold for respiratory stimulation in some patients may approach an arterial Pco_2 of 55 to 60 mmHg, so this level of CO_2 should be attained for the test to be considered positive. A transcutaneous CO_2 monitor may be useful in confirming this level. Furthermore, hypoxia, which can engender cardiac arrhythmia, should be avoided by a 10-min period of ventilation with 100% oxygen before an apnea test.

These clinical criteria for brain death can be supplemented by the documentation of electrocerebral silence on an electroencephalogram[8] or by the absence of cerebral blood flow as shown by a contrast arteriogram, or by radionuclide perfusion scan of the brain.[9]

Donor Screening

While awaiting confirmation of brain death, the potential heart donor can be screened for other criteria of acceptability. In general, these are young, otherwise healthy people. Age is of course a physiologically relative notion, but currently cardiac procurement is generally limited to male donors not older than 40 years and females not older than 45 years.[1,10–12] Most centers will expand these limits to 45 and 50 years, respectively, if coronary angiography can be performed and demonstrates normal coronary anatomy. There should be no evidence of systemic infection or extracranial malignancy. There must be no evidence of active hepatitis, syphilis, tuberculosis, acquired immunodeficiency syndrome (AIDS), or other communicable disease, and no history of illicit intravenous drug use within the previous 10 years. Serum testing for hepatitis and the AIDS antibody have been routine and now, screening for human T lymphotropic virus-1 (HTLV-1) is recommended. Furthermore, patients are excluded if they have known cardiac disease or insulin-dependent diabetes mellitus, and may be excluded with chronic hypertension, and those in whom resuscitation has included prolonged cardiopulmonary resuscitation or the use of intracardiac medications. Most centers are circumspect about those patients requiring "high dose" inotropic support to maintain adequate hemodynamics because these potential donors must be suspected of having less than normal cardiac function.[10,11] In those patients in whom adequate blood pressure is maintained only with high doses of inotropic agents, an echocardiogram can help separate those with depressed cardiac function from those with a good cardiac output in the face of profoundly decreased systemic vascular resistance.[13] Further evaluation of the potential heart donor includes a chest x-ray and an electrocardiogram. Blunt trauma victims frequently lack any external evidence of chest trauma even in the face of significant visceral injury. A chest x-ray is helpful for evaluation of the size and shape of the cardiac silhouette but also for revealing indirect evidence of significant chest trauma. Fractures of the sternum, scapula, or first three ribs all indicate a significant amount of kinetic energy transferred to the thorax and should raise the suspicion of a blunt cardiac injury. Myocardial contusion is the most frequent result of blunt trauma to the heart and the incidence varies according to the methods used to make the diagnosis. In cases where myocardial contusion is considered, cardiac creatine phosphokinase enzyme levels (CPK-MB) should be obtained.

A 12-lead electrocardiogram is performed on all donors and is reassuring when it is normal. Brain injury and herniation alone, however, can induce numerous abnormalities including ST-T changes, bradycardia, junctional rhythm, and sinus tachycardia.[14,15] These are probably related to increased catecholamine levels and may actually be associated with histologic cardiac injury. Arrhythmias are also the most frequent expression of myocardial contusion, with atrial arrhythmias predominating. Whenever there is suspicion of cardiac injury, echocardiography has been found to be very useful. This study allows detection of pericardial fluid, valve function, wall motion, and an estimation of ventricular ejection fraction. The value of echocardiography was recently highlighted in a re-

TABLE 6.2. Screening criteria for cardiac donation.

Age[a]: Males <40 years
           Females <45 years
No prior cardiac disease
No diabetes (insulin-requiring)
No active systemic infection
No potential for transmitting infection
   History of IV drug abuse
   Potential exposure to AIDS
   Serology negative for:
      Hepatitis B
      HIV
      HTLV-1
No malignancy (except primary intracranial)
No evidence for cardiac trauma/dysfunction
   Extensive chest trauma
   Prolonged resuscitation
   Intracardiac injections[b]
   High-dose inotropic support (dopamine >10 µg/kg/min)
   Elevated myocardial fraction of creatine kinase
   Pathologic Q waves on ECG

[a]Some age flexibility is present, especially if coronary angiography can be performed.
[b]Relative contraindication.

port from the UTAH cardiac transplant program.[13] These authors stated that 29% of successfully transplanted hearts would otherwise have been excluded for transplantation using strict clinical criteria if echocardiography had not been employed to evaluate these donors. Acceptable echocardiographic findings included not only a normal echocardiogram, but also a "small" pericardial effusion, equivocal mitral valve prolapse without mitral regurgitation, and isolated "mild" septal hypokinesis. The screening criteria for cardiac donation are summarized in Table 6.2.

Donor Management

Once identified, the heart donor must be managed carefully to maintain adequate organ perfusion and metabolic homeostasis while arrangements are coordinated for cardiac and other organ retrieval. Certain physiological characteristics of the brain dead donor allow predictable responses to foreseeable problems (see Table 6.3). These patients lose their capability of thermal regulation and consequently become cool. This is worsened by the large amounts of volume replacement that is frequently necessary. In addition, hypothermia alone can engender bradycardia. Therefore, efforts should be made to monitor and maintain body temperature above 34°C with a warming blanket. Hypovolemia is frequent in these donors

TABLE 6.3. Donor management problems.

Hypothermia
Hypoxia
  Pulmonary atelectasis
  Neurogenic pulmonary edema
Hypotension
  Dehydration
    Iatrogenic
    Diabetes insipidus
  Vascular collapse
  Cardiac dysfunction
Hypertension
Infection
Acid-base/electrolyte abnormalities
Anemia

for several reasons. Traumatic fluid loss is frequently underestimated and incompletely resuscitated. Furthermore, patients with brain injury are always managed with fluid restriction in an attempt to reduce brain edema and intracranial hypertension.[16] Finally, compromised hypothalamic-pituitary function results in diabetes insipidus with increased urinary volume loss.[17] Additionally, the loss of vasomotor tone results in increased capacitance and relative hypovolemia. For these reasons, fluid resuscitation is frequently necessary and should include generous amounts of a balanced salt solution such as Ringer's lactate solution. Hematocrits should be checked every two to four hours to prevent excessive hemodilution and should be maintained at 25% to 30% with packed red blood cells.

Ideally, cardiac filling pressures are monitored with either a central venous catheter or pulmonary artery catheter. In this case, the central venous pressure or pulmonary capillary wedge pressure should be maintained in the range of 8 to 12 mmHg. If diabetes insipidus is not present, adequate urinary output (0.5 ml/kg per hr) is an indirect measure of adequate volume resuscitation. In the presence of diabetes insipidus, it is useful to treat with aqueous arginine vasopressin. This can be administered as an intermittent intravenous bolus (2–10 U every 2–4 hr) or as a continuous infusion with titration to maintain urine output less than 200 ml/hr. Blood pressure in the brain dead donor can be extremely labile and maintenance of cardiovascular stability is at times difficult.[18,19] Loss of vasomotor tone and severe hypotension are frequent. If volume resuscitation is not sufficient to raise perfusion pressures significantly (systolic blood pressure >90 mmHg), then vasopressor support is indicated. Dopamine is the preferred agent in potential multiorgan donors because of its preferential effect of increasing renal perfusion at low doses (3–5 μg/kg per min). Intermittent hypotensive periods before cardiac procurement can result in postoperative graft dysfunction, particularly if these periods of hypotension and relative ischemia are prolonged.[11] At the other end of the blood pressure spectrum, hypothalamic stimulation and extensive catecholamine discharge can result from intracranial hypertension and engender severe arterial hypertension. This greatly increased systemic vascular resistance increases cardiac work and decreases cardiac output. Also, this increase in sympathetic tone can cause subendocardial ischemia and ventricular arrhythmias. This may be a frequent cause of unexplained cardiac dysfunction in donors with negative cardiac histories and absence of chest trauma. Within minutes of the acute adrenergic discharge, a substantial amount of myocardial degeneration, subendocardial hemorrhage, and myocardial necrosis can occur.[20,21] Important hypertension should therefore be approached in a determined manner and managed with cautious afterload reduction using sodium nitroprusside.

Adequate blood gas exchange is usually a straightforward intensive care management process. Mechanical ventilation with a volume-controlled respirator is the rule and tidal volumes are typically 10 to 15 ml/kg. However, many brain-injured patients will have been managed with hyperventilation protocols in an effort to decrease intracranial pressure by inducing hypocarbia.[16] When brain death is declared in these patients, the focus should more appropriately shift toward maintenance of normocarbia because the alkalosis resulting from hyperventilation shifts the oxyhemoglobin dissociation curve to the right, thereby decreasing tissue availability of oxygen. Oxygenation should be maintained with a goal of keeping a PO_2 of 80 mmHg or greater or an oxygen saturation (SO_2 of 92% or better). In general, this can be achieved with an inspired oxygen fraction (FIO_2 of 40% or less) but associated pulmonary contusion, atelectasis, fluid overload, or "shock lung" can decrease oxygen exchange and increase shunting such that higher oxygen concentrations and positive end expiratory pressure (PEEP) are necessary. A problem specific to the brain-injured patient is that of "neurogenic pulmonary edema", which is similarly managed with diuresis and appropriate FIO_2 and PEEP.[19] The nursing care of these intubated brain-dead donors is of prime importance. Aggressive, frequent endotracheal irrigation and suctioning are necessary to control secretions and prevent atelectasis and pneumonia. The patients should be turned frequently if tolerated hemodynamically. A patent nasogastric tube should be maintained to avoid gastric distention and aspiration. Broad spectrum antibiotics are used empirically in these patients as prophylaxis against iatrogenic sepsis. With careful attention to monitoring of the details of donor homeostasis, ideal conditions can be maintained.

Myocardial Preservation

During the last decade, one key factor that has substantially improved the surgical outlook for patients with cardiac disease has been better operative preservation of the myocardium, and in particular, utilization of cold cardioplegic techniques. It is only natural that these techniques have been extended to the preservation of the donor heart, both at the time of harvesting and at the time of implantation. The basis of myocardial preservation is the rapid induction of cardiac arrest and hypothermia with sparing of the high-energy phosphate stores and maintaining the heart in this cold, flaccid, and nonworking state before reperfusion. Most cardioplegic solutions (see Chapter 7, Table 7.1) utilize high concentrations of potassium to achieve pharmacologic arrest of the heart and to prevent tonic cardiac contractions or fibrillation (which by requiring energy would deplete high-energy phosphate stores) during cooling.

Oxygen consumption and metabolic rate fall in a linear fashion with body temperature, and tolerance to ischemia is extended by hypothermia.[22] As has been confirmed by the relationship between temperature and functional recovery after arrest,[23] there is excellent protection of the myocardium at between 5° and 20°C using cold crystalloid cardioplegia. Cessation of cardiac activity with these solutions is of utmost importance because 80% of the myocardial oxygen consumption arises from mechanical work.[24] Myocardial cooling via the aortic root and coronary perfusion is enhanced by the addition of topical cooling with large amounts of 4°C-balanced electrolyte solutions that wash out the pericardial cavity at the time of cardiectomy. With this most commonly used myocardial preservation and cardiac harvesting technique, the donor heart is transported in a cold environment to prevent premature warming.

Other less commonly and intermittently used cardiac preservation methods have included an autoperfused heart-lung preparation and core-cooling on cardiopulmonary bypass.[25,26] The major advantage of the latter method has been to facilitate and reduce the harvesting time of multiple organ procurements by providing a relatively bloodless operative field.

Future Directions and Conclusions

The primary limitation to heart transplantation is the limited number of donor hearts available for transplantation. It is estimated that as many as 15,000 patients per year could benefit from heart transplantation, yet only around 10% of this group are likely to receive a donor heart. For this reason, multiple approaches have been taken in an attempt to increase the donor pool.

Donor age has been gradually expanded, and as previously mentioned, it is now routine to accept male donors to the age of 40 years and females to the age of 45 years. These upper limits have been expanded further for desperately ill patients on waiting lists. Based on recent data, the expansion of the donor age criteria does not appear to have impacted recipient outcome.[27] Whether further donor age expansion can occur is a regular topic of debate and is advocated by several groups.

A certain percentage of donor hearts are deemed unacceptable because of ventricular dysfunction. Recent evidence suggests that major hormonal levels and specifically thyroid hormone levels are acutely reduced during and after brain death.[28] Futhermore, the repletion of thyroid hormone in these donors may improve cardiac performance.[29]

It is hoped that multiple factors may improve the availability of donor organs. Studies investigating further expansion of donor age and other criteria are currently in progress. A more aggressive approach to patients having cerebrovascular catastrophes including not only optimal protection of the central nervous system but protection of other organ systems (e.g., blood pressure control, catecholamine toxicity) may have positive effects whether or not brain death occurs ultimately. Based on encouraging early results, a careful assessment of the donor's metabolic and hormonal status may prove fruitful in reducing the number of discarded organs. Finally, the ultimate means of increasing available hearts and other organs for transplantation will be through intensive and broad-scale public and professional education programs.

References

1. Heck CF, Shumway SJ, Kaye MP. The registry of the International Society for Heart Transplantation: sixth official report—1989. *J Heart Transplant.* 1989;8:271.
2. Sadler AM, Sadler BL, Statson EB. The Uniform Anatomical Gift Act. *JAMA.* 1968;206:2501.
3. Black PM: Brain death. *N Engl J Med.* 1978;299:338.
4. Powner DJ. The diagnosis of brain death in the adult patient. *J Intens Care Med.* 1987;2:181.
5. Pallis C. Prognostic significance of a dead brain stem. *Br Med J.* 1981;282:533.
6. Ivan LP: Spinal reflexes in cerebral death. *Neurology.* 1973;23:650.
7. Ropper AH, Kennedy SK, Russell L. Apnea testing in the diagnosis of brain death. *J Neurosurg.* 1981;55:942.
8. Powner DJ, Fromm GH. The electroencephalogram in the determination of brain death. *N Engl J Med.* 1979;300:502.
9. Greitz T, Gordon E, Kolmodin G, Widen L. Aortocranial and carotid angiography in determination of brain death. *Neuroradiology.* 1973;5:13.
10. Emery RW, Cork RC, Levinson MM, et al. The cardiac donor: a six year experience. *Ann Thorac Surg.* 1986;41:356.
11. Griepp RB, Stinson EB, Clark DA, et al. The cardiac donor. *Surg Gynecol Obstet.* 1971;133:792.
12. Copeland JG: Cardiac transplantation. *Curr Probl Cardiol.* 1988;13:159.
13. Gilbert EM, Krieger SK, Murray JL, et al. Echocardiographic evaluation of potential cardiac transplant donors. *J Thorac Cardiovasc Surg.* 1988;95:1003.
14. Fentz V, Gormsen J. Electrocardiographic patterns in patients with cerebrovascular accidents. *Circulation.* 1962;25:22.
15. Novitzky D, Wicomb WN, Cooper DKC, et al. Electrocardiographic, hemodynamic and endocrine changes occuring during experimental brain death in the chacma baboon. *J Heart Transplant.* 1984;4:63.

16. Lewin W. Factors in the mortality of closed head injuries. *Br Med J.* 1953;1:1239.
17. Walker AE. Practical considerations in the treatment of head injuries. *Neurology.* 1951;1:75.
18. Frilman NF, Jeffers WA. Effect of progressive sympathectomy on hypertension produced by increased intracranial pressure. *Am J Physiol.* 1940;128:662.
19. Ducker TB. Increased intracranial pressure and pulmonary edema. I. Clinical study of 11 patients. *J Neurosurg.* 1968;28:112.
20. Marion DW, Ricardo S, Thompson ME. Subarachnoid hemorrhage and the heart. *Neurosurgery.* 1986;18:101.
21. McLeod AA, Neil-Dwyer G, Meyer CHA, Richardson PL, Cruickshank J, Bartlett J. Cardiac sequelea of acute head injury. *Br Heart J.* 1982;47:221.
22. Bigelow WG, Lindsay WK, Greenwood WF. Hypothermia. Its possible role in cardiac surgery: an investigation of factors governing survival in dogs at low body temperatures. *Ann Surg.* 1950;132:849.
23. Hearse DJ, Stewart DA, Braimbridge MV. Cellular protection during myocardial ischemia: the development and characterization of a procedure for the induction of reversible ischemic arrest. *Circulation.* 1976;54:193.
24. Braunwald E. The determinants of myocardial oxygen consumption. *Physiologist.* 1969;12:65.
25. Adachi H, Fraser CD, Kontos GJ, et al. Autoperfused working heart-lung preparation versus hypothermia cardiopulmonary preservation for transplantation. *J Heart Transplant.* 1987;6:253.
26. Hardesty RL, Griffith BP. Procurement for combined heart-lung transplantation. *J Thorac Cardiovasc Surg.* 1985;89:795.
27. Mulvagh SL, Thornton B, Frazier OH, et al. The older cardiac transplant donor. Relation to graft function and recipient survival longer than 6 years. *Circulation.* 1989;80(suppl):III–126.
28. Gifford RPM, Weaver AS, Burg JE, et al. Thyroid hormone levels in heart and kidney cadaver donors. *J Heart Transplant.* 1986;5:249.
29. Novitsky D, Cooper DKC, Zuhdi N. The physiological management of cardiac transplant donors and recipients using triiodothyronine. *Transplant Proc.* 1988;20:803.

7
Operative Techniques and Early Postoperative Care in Cardiac Transplantation

ADNAN COBANOGLU

Although heart transplantation has become a popular therapeutic modality in only the last decade, the technical groundwork started in the early 1900s and spanned more than 60 years (see Chapter 1), ultimately leading to the first successful clinical orthotopic allograft heart transplantation in 1967.[1-7] In addition to decades of work refining the operative technique, particularly over the last two decades, significant improvements in cardiac anesthesia and conduct of extracorporeal circulation, and better myocardial preservation techniques have all contributed to excellent operative outcome in heart transplantation. Today it is not unrealistic to expect a surgical mortality of well below 10%.

Timing and Logistics of Donor-Recipient Operations

With the scarcity of donors and the tremendous demand for organs, organ procurement is performed at distant donor sites and multiple teams are involved in the harvesting of multiple organs. Close attention to timing of recipient and donor operations in heart transplantation has never been more important. In order to achieve best functional results with the transplanted cardiac allograft, the total ischemic time should be kept to a minimum.[8,9] Most centers have tried to keep this period to less than 4 hours, which translates into 3 hours of total transport time (approximately 1500 miles of air travel) and an hour of implantation. For severely ill, hemodynamically unstable patients who otherwise might not survive, these time limits are generally extended. With an increasing number of recipients who have had previous open heart surgery (38% of cases at Oregon Health Sciences University), one has to allow additional time for a meticulous cardiac dissection and have the recipient ready for cardiectomy as soon as the donor heart arrives. If one is to err in timing, it is best to have more time for the recipient in order not to have to rush the anesthesia and sternotomy in these patients because they are usually critically ill.

The Donor Cardiectomy

Since multiple teams are usually involved in the donor operation, the sequence of events should be collectively reviewed before starting the procedure and intraoperatively all moves should be made in close collaboration with other teams.[10,11] It is appropriate that the cardiac surgeon take the leadership role in the intraoperative management of the donor and direct the fluid and drug therapy as necessary. In extreme hemodynamic instability refractory to therapeutic maneuvers, the heart would take priority over other organs and would be harvested after notifying other teams working on the liver, kidneys, and so on.

It is desirable to have good control of the donor's hemodynamic status, which can be assisted by the use of large-bore intravenous lines, an arterial pressure monitor line and a central venous catheter. The cardiac surgery team may have to insert some of these lines before surgery in smaller hospitals with limited personnel and expertise in donor management.

The heart and other organs are approached through a long mid-line incision from the suprasternal notch to the symphysis pubis. The pericardium is incised and the mid-line incision is deepened in the area where the central tendon of the diaphragm fuses with its inferior surface. After pericardiotomy, the heart is carefully examined for evidence of contusion, coronary artery disease, valvular heart disease, or congenital anomaly. Sanguinous or serosanguinous effusion upon entry into the pericardial space might indicate myocardial trauma and injury.

Once the decision is made to use the heart, the ascending aorta and inferior vena cava are dissected free and controlled with tapes. The pulmonary artery is dissected free to its bifurcation. The superior vena cava is controlled with two heavy silk ties and dissected off the right pulmonary artery underneath it (Fig. 7.1). Further dissection that might disturb the hemodynamic stability is not done and the circulation is supported while the abdominal organs are harvested. Just before harvesting of organs, 30,000 units of heparin are administered intravenously.

Proper myocardial preservation at the time of harvesting is obviously of utmost importance for good cardiac function in the recipient after transplantation. Methods that are used on a daily basis in open heart procedures are used during cardiac harvest and include hypothermia and cardioplegic arrest of the heart. Selective cardiac hypothermia decreases oxygen consumption significantly and this is further enhanced by chemical cardioplegia, since 80% of myocardial oxygen consumption arises from mechanical work.[12,13] For this purpose we prepare a cold crystalloid potassium cardioplegia solution (Table 7.1). This solution is kept at 3° to 4°C before administration.

When harvesting is begun, the superior vena cava is doubly ligated and divided between ligatures, then the inferior vena cava is clamped right above the diaphragm. The heart is allowed to beat and empty for a few seconds, then the ascending aorta is cross-clamped at innominate artery take-off and the cardioplegic solution (1000 ml) is infused into the aortic root. The right

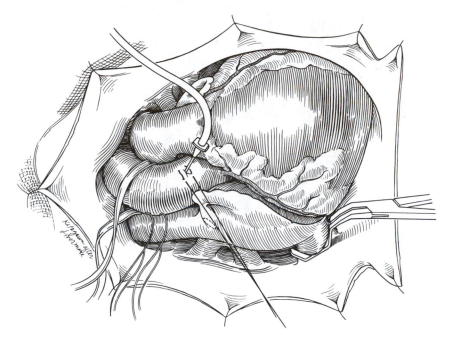

FIGURE 7.1. Donor cardiectomy. The ascending aorta, inferior vena cava, and pulmonary artery are dissected free. The superior vena cava is controlled with silk ties.

inferior pulmonary vein and the inferior vena cava are transected immediately (Fig. 7.2). During cardioplegic solution infusion, approximately 8 to 10 L of ice-cold physiologic solution is used for topical cooling and bathing the heart. The aorta is transected at the origin of the innominate artery and the main pulmonary artery at its bifurcation (Fig. 7.3). All pulmonary veins are transected and the specimen is removed (Fig. 7.4), rinsed in two basins of balanced electrolyte solution, and packed for transport. Before transplantation the donor heart is prepared for implantation by incising across and connecting the pulmonary veins and trimming the excess left atrial tissue.

TABLE 7.1. Oregon Health Sciences University cardioplegic solution.

Basic solution	Ringer's solution
K$^+$(mEq/L)	25
Na$^+$(mEq/L)	152
Ca^{2+}(mEq/L)	405
HCO$_3$(mEq/L)	25
Glucose (mg/dl)	0.2
pH	7.8
Osmolality (mosmol)	360

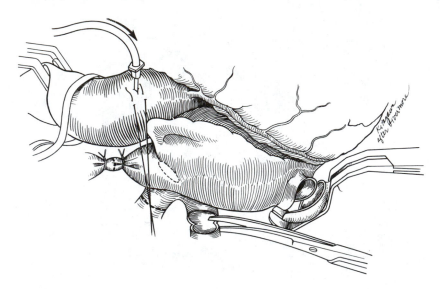

FIGURE 7.2. Donor cardiectomy. The right inferior pulmonary vein and the inferior vena cava are transected.

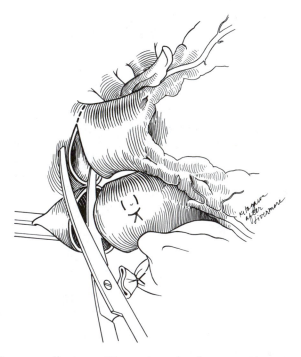

FIGURE 7.3. Donor cardiectomy. The aorta and pulmonary artery are transected.

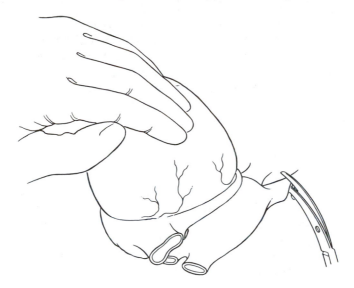

FIGURE 7.4. Donor cardiectomy. All pulmonary veins are transected and the heart is removed.

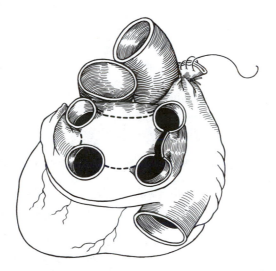

FIGURE 7.5. Donor heart preparation. Before transplantation the donor pulmonary veins are connected with incisions as shown, and excess tissue removed. The superior vena cava tie is reinforced.

The superior vena cava tie is reinforced with a circumferential 4-0 polypropylene suture, as well as the cardioplegia administration site in the ascending aorta (Fig. 7.5). The interatrial septum is inspected for presence of a patent foramen ovale; if present, this is fixed to prevent a significant right-to-left shunt that might result from temporary right ventricular dysfunction, poor compliance, and elevated right atrial pressures.

The Recipient Operation

The patient comes into the operating room after having received all immunosuppressive drugs and prophylactic antibiotics (see Appendix I). If a distant donor procurement is to be done, the patient is not anesthetized until the donor heart is visualized and examined. Timing is more critical when the donor is in the transplant hospital or within close proximity. In these cases, particularly if the recipient has had prior cardiac surgery, the recipient is anesthetized, prepped, and draped, and all is ready to make the incision once the donor heart is inspected. The recipient should have one or two large-bore peripheral intravenous catheters, a radial artery catheter, and a left internal jugular vein catheter. Strict sterile technique must be observed at all times during catheter placement. In critically ill patients who have hemodynamic instability, or when weaning from cardiopulmonary bypass is expected to be difficult, a balloon-tipped, flow-directed pulmonary artery catheter should be placed. This catheter can be preserved during cardiectomy and then replaced just before completion of right atrial anastomosis, and before pulmonary artery anastomosis. Postoperatively in patients who have demonstrated instability, this catheter has been invaluable in assessment and management of hemodynamics.

The recipient's heart is approached through a median sternotomy, the pericardial cavity is entered, and the pericardial edges are sutured to wound stockinettes. The aorta and superior and inferior vena cavae are circumferentially controlled with umbilical tapes. Tourniquets are passed onto caval tapes. After systemic heparinization (3 mg/kg), the aorta is cannulated as distal as possible below the origin of the innominate artery. The superior and inferior vena cavae are cannulated through pursestrings placed on the right atrium close to the interatrial groove.

The recipient's heart should not be excised until the donor heart arrives at the operating room. At that point cardiopulmonary bypass is started, superior and inferior caval tourniquets are tightened down, and the ascending aorta is cross-clamped after the heart empties in a few beats. The core temperature is usually taken down to 26°C.

The native heart is excised starting with an incision at the base of the right atrial appendage on the right lateral wall of the right atrium and close to the atrioventricular junction (Fig. 7.6). A small incision in the interatrial septum is made and a coronary suction catheter is introduced into the left side to decompress the left heart and facilitate the excision (Fig. 7.7). The right

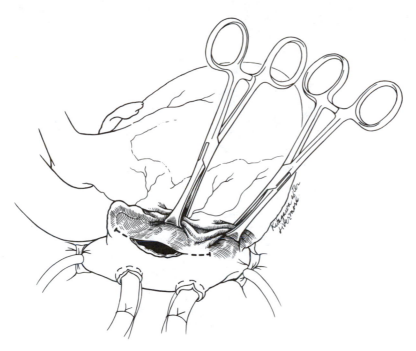

FIGURE 7.6. Recipient cardiectomy. The native heart is excised starting with an incision at the base of the right artrial appendage on the right lateral wall of the right atrium.

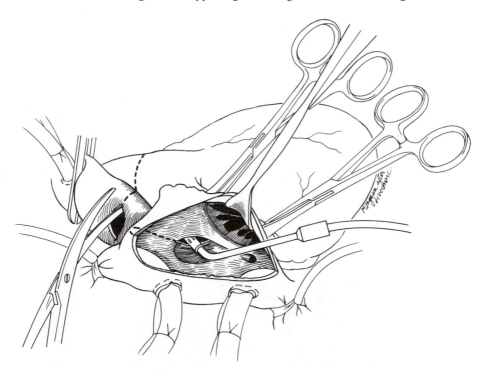

FIGURE 7.7. Recipient cardiectomy. A small incision in the interatrial septum is made and a coronary suction catheter is introduced into the left side.

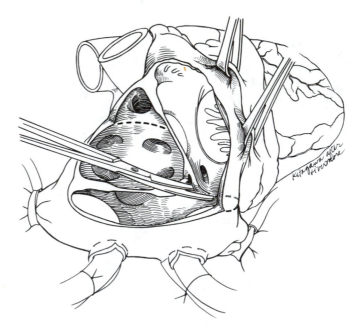

FIGURE 7.8. Recipient cardiectomy. The right atrial incision is carried downward toward the left side and across the interatrial septum while making sure that the coronary sinus is left on the specimen side and that most of the interatrial septum is left behind.

atrial incision is carried downward and toward the left side and across the interatrial septum, making sure that the coronary sinus is left on the specimen side and that most of the interatrial septum is left behind (Fig. 7.8). The aorta and the main pulmonary artery are divided close to the corresponding semilunar valves. The incision in the right atrium and the interatrial septum is carried on leftward to the dome of the left atrium and toward the base of the left atrial appendage. The left lateral wall of the left atrium is the last area that is incised, making sure that an adequate cuff of atrial tissue remains in front of the pulmonary veins for suturing without causing pulmonary venous obstruction (Fig. 7.9).

The prepared donor heart is sutured starting with the left upper corner of the left atrial cuff and the base of the left atrial appendage of the donor heart. One arm of a 54-inch long double-armed 3-0 polypropylene suture is carried downward in an over-and-over fashion toward the diaphragmatic surface of the left atrium and then up to the mid-portion of the interatrial septum (Fig. 7.10). The second arm of the suture is carried in a similar manner across the dome of the left atrium to the interatrial septum and this suture is secured on the outside of the left atrium (Fig. 7.11).

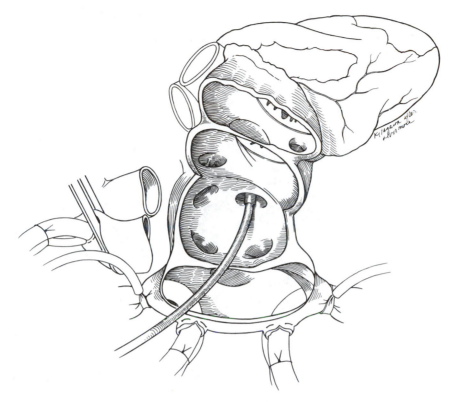

FIGURE 7.9. Recipient cardiectomy. The aorta and the main pulmonary artery are divided. The incision in the right atrium and the interatrial septum is carried on leftward. The left lateral wall of the left atrium is the last area that is incised.

The right free wall of the right atrium is incised obliquely starting at the lateral wall of the inferior vena cava up toward the base of the right atrial appendage. It is important to avoid the sinoatrial node and to leave enough of a cuff anteriorly to enable suturing without damage to the node or internodal pathways in the area of crista terminalis. A second 54-inch polypropylene suture is used to anastamose the donor right atrium to the right atrial cuff. This suture is started in the mid-portion of the interatrial septum and overlays the left atrial suture line to some degree. One arm is carried around clockwise to the right lateral wall of the right atrium and the second arm is carried around counterclockwise. This suture is secured on the lateral wall of the right atrium (Fig. 7.12.)

Although some have advocated performing the aortic anastomosis next and then removing the cross-clamp, the approach at Oregon Health Sciences University has been to attach the donor and recipient pulmonary arteries in a quiet, bloodless field while the clamp is still on. The anastomosis is started on the left lateral side of the arteries and carried around

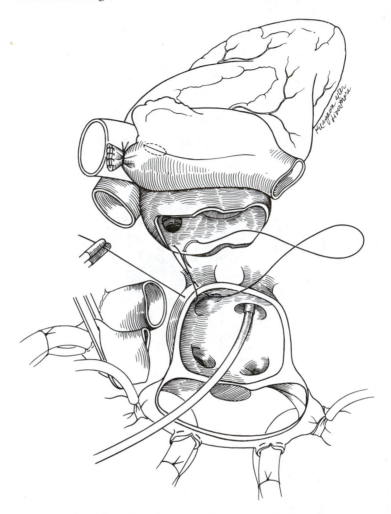

FIGURE 7.10. Implantation. Suturing starts in between the left upper corner of the left atrial cuff and the base of the left atrial appendage of the donor heart.

with a double-armed 4-0 polypropylene suture. This suture is left untied anteriorly to use later during the cardiac resuscitation period (Fig. 7.12C).

The aortae are sutured with a double-armed 4-0 polypropylene suture in a similar manner, starting at the left side of the aorta and moving in both directions. The suture is tied down anteriorly. During this anastomosis the patient is rewarmed to 37°C. A separate pursestring is placed at

FIGURE 7.11. Implantation. A, The suture is carried in a similar manner across the dome of the left atrium to the interatrial septum and B, this suture is secured on the outside of the left atrium.

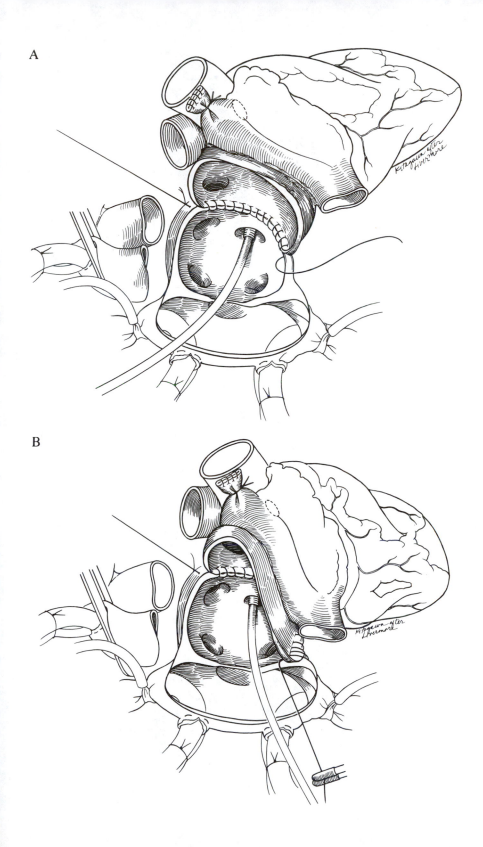

A

B

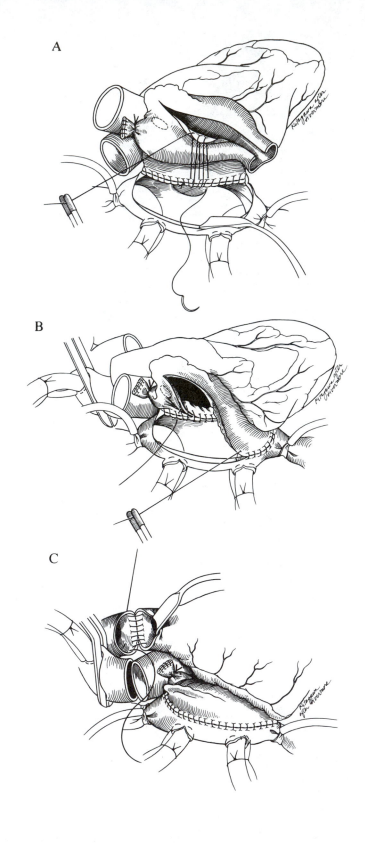

A

B

C

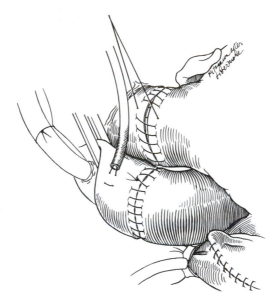

FIGURE 7.13. Implantation. After anastamosis of the pulmonary arteries, the aortae are sutured in a similar manner. A separate pursestring is placed at the highest point of the ascending aorta to introduce a large-bore needle to vent intracardiac air.

the highest point of the ascending aorta to introduce a large-bore needle to vent intracardiac air during ejection (Fig. 7.13). Ventricular pacing electrodes are placed in the anterior wall of the right ventricle. The heart is electrically fibrillated while the ascending aorta is vented and the aortic cross-clamp is removed. Caval tapes and tourniquets are removed; all intracardiac air is evacuated with aspiration of the right superior pulmonary vein and the left ventricular apex. The heart is defibrillated while the ascending aortic vent is still open. Varying amounts of time (usually 15–20 min) are allowed for the donor heart to recover while still on by-pass. Quite frequently a continuous intravenous infusion of isoproterenol (0.005–0.01 pg/kg per min) is started to promote sinus rhythm and a heart rate of 100 to 110 beats/min. Infusions of dopamine, epinephrine, and ni-

←

FIGURE 7.12. Implantation. A, The right free wall of the right atrium is incised obliquely starting at the lateral wall of the inferior vena cava up toward the base of the right atrial appendage. B, A second suture is used to anastamose the donor right atrium to the right atrial cuff, starting in the mid-portion of the interatrial septum and overlays the left atrial suture line to some degree. One arm is carried around clockwise to the right lateral wall of the right atrium and the second arm is carried around counterclockwise. This suture is secured on the lateral wall of the right atrium. C, The donor and recipient pulmonary arteries are starting on the left side with running suture.

troprusside are added as necessary in cases where right or left ventricular dysfunction or both are likely.

Once at 37°C, with normal sinus rhythm and good contractility, the patient is weaned off cardiopulmonary bypass. Protamine is administered to counter-effect the heparin. Decannulation and sternotomy closure are carried out in a routine manner. Two mediastinal drainage catheters and pleural catheters (if these cavities have been entered) are used. The usual cardiac implantation time is 45 to 50 min and cardiopulmonary bypass time is 90 to 120 min.

Quite clearly, during harvesting of the donor heart and other organs and preparation of the recipient and the actual transplantation operation, there are many little details that must be meticulously attended to in order to secure successful outcome. Precise coordination, collaboration, and communication are never more important.

Reoperations

Most cardiac transplant services treat an increasing number of patients who have had prior cardiac operations due to coronary artery disease, valvular heart disease, or congenital heart defects.

If patients have been on sodium warfarin or heparin preoperatively, consideration should be given to using fresh frozen plasma in the pump prime solution.

Importance of meticulous attention to hemostasis at the time of sternotomy cannot be overemphasized. It is better to stop bleeding on the way in rather than on the way out. Electrocautery is used liberally throughout the procedure. Dissection is carried out to allow enough exposure of the right heart and the ascending aorta to cannulate and initiate cardiopulmonary bypass. In cases where an internal mammary graft is present, only minimal dissection is performed over the left heart. The left-sided dissection and separation of the aorta from the pulmonary artery can be performed once on bypass. The latter is easier once cardiectomy is done because the plane between the two vessels can be better identified. If one encounters multiple proximal vein graft anastamoses, the aorta is transected at the usual level and the proximal sites remaining on the aorta are oversewn. If there are dense adhesions in between the heart and pericardium or the adjacent lung due to felt pledgets, automatic defibrillator pads, electrodes, and so forth, thereby making dissection inordinately difficult, these could be left behind on the pericardium.

After discontinuation of cardiopulmonary bypass, one must be cautious in using blood and blood products. The pulmonary vascular resistance and right ventricular function are delicately balanced in most cases, and overzealous use of blood, fresh frozen plasma, or platelet infusions could tip this balance unfavorably. These should be given only if bleeding is truly excessive.

TABLE 7.2. Intravenous agents used in the immediate postoperative period.

Adrenergic agents	a-Effect	B-Effect
Dobutamine (2–30 mg/kg/min)	+	+ + + +
Dopamine (2–30 mg/kg/min)	+ +	+ + +
Epinephrine (0.025–0.25 mg/kg/min)	+ + +	+ + +
Isoproterenol (0.005–0.08 mg/kg/min)	–	+ + + +
Vasodilators	Venous	Arterial
Nitroglycerin (0.3–6 mg/kg/min)	+ + +	+
Nitroprusside (0.3–8 mg/kg/min)	+ +	+ + +

Early Postoperative Care

Hemodynamic Monitoring and Support

The most common cause of hospital death early after cardiac transplantation is acute right ventricular failure or global biventricular dysfunction with low output syndrome. In cases of early postoperative left or biventricular dysfunction, the cause is likely to be myocardial stunning due to ischemia or suboptimal myocardial preservation and usually resolves within 48 to 72 hours. Conversely, patients with prior pulmonary hypertension and increased pulmonary vascular resistance are more likely postoperatively to develop right ventricular dysfunction. The therapeutic manipulations for these two scenarios may require vastly different approaches, which can be greatly facilitated by the use of a balloon-tipped, flow-directed pulmonary artery catheter (now used routinely because of the higher risk patients and extended ischemic times). Ischemic injury results in myocardial edema, decreased compliance, and in more severe cases a reduction in systolic function. Both left and right ventricular filling pressures are elevated[14] and it is not infrequent that despite this, additional volume is required to optimize preload (sarcomere length) to improve cardiac output. If filling pressures are already excessive and poor cardiac output persists, a combination of inotropic support and vasodilator therapy is indicated.[15-19] In most cases small doses of dopamine or dobutamine are adequate to maintain cardiac output. In patients with elevated systemic vascular resistance, small doses of sodium nitroprusside can be added (Table 7.2).

In patients with acute right ventricular dysfunction secondary to pulmonary hypertension, the state of the heart is similar to that seen with acute right ventricular infarction. The right ventricle is dilated with impaired contractility, right ventricular output is inadequate to fill the left ventricle, and hypotension ensues.[20] In contrast with right ventricular infarction, the pulmonary vasculature is not normal and volume expansion results in additional distension of the right ventricle (which likely has some degree of preservation injury), and further deterioration of hemodynamics. In this case, the primary therapy is inotropic support. If blood pressure can be maintained, systemic vasodilators may be of some benefit for their effects on the pulmonary vasculature. In addition, some groups have used prostaglandin E infusions in this circumstance for more selective pulmonary vasodilation.[21]

Isoproterenol, a direct-acting beta agonist, is a commonly used drug. It increases the heart rate, causes peripheral vasodilation, and augments the cardiac output substantially. It is not unusual to continue an infusion of isoproterenol for 2 to 4 days postoperatively. In cases where heart rate is refractory to pharmacologic maneuvers, epicardial atrial and ventricular pacing is used to optimize heart rate.

When pharmacologic measures are inadequate in dealing with the low output state, a means of mechanical circulatory assist becomes necessary. The intraaortic balloon pump (IABP) is often extremely effective when the cardiac index is 1.0 to 1.8 L/m^2 per m in secondary to biventricular dysfunction. IABP reduces both left ventricular afterload and preload with eventual reduction in myocardial oxygen demand. It augments the coronary blood flow by 30% to 35% by increasing diastolic pressure and improvement in zonal myocardial perfusion. It produces an average increase in cardiac output of 20% to 25%.[22,23] In extreme refractory cases of low cardiac output, one might have to resort to the use of unilateral or bilateral ventricular assist systems and/or retransplantation.

Protective Isolation and Infection Control

Based on the initial Stanford experience, most centers still use protective isolation to varying degrees. Table 7.3 presents the results of a survey of west coast cardiac transplant centers and their current isolation practices. It is important to emphasize that there are currently no supporting data regarding the use of protective isolation in this patient population yet there are studies suggesting the lack of benefit for these procedures.[24]

Other infection control measures include the rapid removal of intravenous, intraarterial, and bladder catheters and early extubation to prevent catheter and pulmonary infections. Vigorous pulmonary toilet and early ambulation are also used to prevent pulmonary atelectasis. Frequent surveillance cultures and prophylactic antibiotics to cover common skin bacteria are used in most centers covering the time that catheters are in place. Finally, some centers use prophylactic trimethoprim sulfa and cytomegalovirus globulin for patients at risk.

Immunosuppression

Immunosuppression is covered extensively in Chapter 9; however, several features deserve brief comment here. The immunosuppressive protocols used at Oregon Health Sciences University are presented in Appen-

TABLE 7.3. Protective isolation procedures.

	Private room	Hand washing	Gloves	Gowns	Marks	Shoe covers	Hats
Intensive Care Unit							
OHSU[a]	+	+	+	+	+	−	−
Center 1	+	+	+	+	+	+	+
Center 2	+	+	+	+	+	+	+
Center 3	+	+	−	−	−	−	−
Center 4	+	+	−	−	+	+	−
Center 5	+	+	−	+	−	−	−
Center 6	+	+	+	+	+	+	+
Ward							
OHSU	+	+	−	−	+	−	−
Center 1	+	+	+	−	+	+	−
Center 2	+	+	−	−	+	+	−
Center 3	+	+	−	−	−	−	−
Center 4	+	+	−	−	+	−	−
Center 5	+	+	−	−	−	−	−
Center 6	+	+	+	−	+	−	−

[a]OHSU = Oregon Health Sciences University.

dix II. In general, after loading doses of immunosuppression are given preoperatively, all immunosuppression at this institution is administered by intravenous route in the first 48 to 72 hours to ensure adequate bio-availability. By administering cyclosporine (2.5–3.0 mg/kg) by continuous infusion over 24 hours, therapeutic levels are achieved rapidly and fluctuations are minimal during this time period. No evidence of excessive renal toxicity has been noted using this protocol. Most transplant centers, however, administer cyclosporine via the nasogastric tube immediately postoperatively.

In patients who have moderate or severe renal insufficiency in the immediate or early postoperative period, cyclosporine can be avoided by using the monoclonal antibody to CD3, OKT3. Cyclosporine is then instituted on postoperative day 11 (see Appendix II).

Miscellaneous Medical Care

Ventilator support with a volume-cycled mechanical respirator is provided for 12 to 24 hours with early extubation if possible. With careful monitoring of fluid status and arterial oxygenation, most patients can be weaned from the respirator within 24 hours of the transplant operation. After cardiac transplantation patients usually require 3 to 4 days in the cardiac recovery room (intensive care), another week to 10 days on the hospital ward, and are usually ready for hospital discharge by postoperative day 12 to 14.

Most patients undergoing cardiac transplantation have intravascular as well as interstitial volume expansion. In addition, patients often receive fluid and blood products intraoperatively. As the peripheral vasodilatory effects of anesthesia wear off, to a variable degree volume is shunted centrally, raising cardiac filling pressures. The maintenance of adequate urine output to compensate for excess volume is therefore required but can be further complicated by the renal vasoconstrictive properties of cyclosporine.[25] In patients refractory to large doses of intravenous furosemide, intravenous ethacrinic acid in modest doses (50–100 mg) may be effective in the early postoperative period. Following daily weights is extremely important in deciding on the degree of diuresis.

Rehabilitation and Patient Education

All patients undergoing cardiac transplantation, by the nature of their underlying disease, have been sedentary and have suffered severe physical deconditioning. Most centers are therefore aggressive in instituting physical therapy early postcardiac transplantation in an attempt to begin to reverse the deconditioning process. It is not unusual at Oregon Health Sciences University for patients to be ambulating while still in the intensive care setting, and riding a stationary bicycle under supervision 4 to 5 days after the transplant operation. Physical therapy is continued for several weeks after transplantation.

Finally, patient education is instituted as soon as possible while patients are recovering from the operation. No patient is allowed to be discharged without first demonstrating a working understanding of cardiac transplant physiology (as it relates to exercise and daily activities), rejection and infection surveillance, and a complete understanding of the patient's medication dosages, schedules, and side effects.

Conclusions

Over a period of two decades, significant advances have been made in all aspects of cardiac transplantation, including better stabilization of transplant candidates in heart failure, advances in immunosuppression manipulation, and anesthesia in patients with severely compromised circulations. Refinement in operative techniques and better myocardial preservation methods have enabled rapid recovery of the transplanted heart and excellent graft function in most cases in the immediate postoperative period. With continued improvement in postoperative care and medical management of early graft dysfunction, hospital mortality after cardiac transplantation has continued to decline and approach levels enjoyed by routine cardiovascular surgery.

References

1. Carrel A. The transplantation of organs: a preliminary communication. *JAMA*. 1905;45:1645–1650.
2. Guthrie CC. Survival of engrafted tissues. *JAMA*. 1910;54:831–834.
3. Mann FC, Priestley JT, Markowitz J, et al. Transplantation of the intact mammalian heart. *Arch Surg*. 1933;26:219–221.
4. Downie HG. Homotransplantation of the dog heart. *Arch Surg*. 1953;66:624–628.
5. Berman EF, Goldberg M, Akman L. Experimental replacement of the heart in the dog. *Transplant Bull*. 1958;5:10–15.
6. Lower RR, Shumway NE. Studies on orthotopic homotransplantation of the canine heart. *Surg Forum*. 1960;11:18–22.
7. Barnard CN. The operation. A human cardiac transplant: an interim report of a successful operation performed at Groote Schurr Hospital, Cape Town. *S Afr Med J*. 1967;41:1271.
8. Griepp RB, Stinson EB, Clark DA, et al. The cardiac donor. *Surg Gynecol Obstet*. 1971;133:792.
9. Billingham ME, Baumgartner WA, Watson DC, et al. Distant heart procurement for human transplantation: ultrastructural studies. *Circulation*. 1980;62(suppl I):1–11.
10. Goldman MH, Shapiro R, Capehart J, et al. Cardiac procurement in the multiple organ donor. *Transplant Proc*. 1984;16:231–234.
11. Hardesty LH, Griffith BP, Trento A, Starzl TE, Bahnson HT. Multiple cadaveric organ procurement for transplantation with emphasis on the heart. *Surg Rounds*. July 1985, 20–34.
12. Buckberg GD, Brazle JR, Nelson RH, et al. Studies on the effects of hypothermia on regional myocardial flow and metabolism during cardiopulmonary bypass. I. The adequately perfused, beating and arrested heart. *J Thorac Cardiovasc Surg*. 1977;73:87–94.
13. Braunwald E. The determinants of myocardial oxygen consumption. *Physiologist*. 1969;12:65–93.
14. Hosenpud JD, Norman DJ, Cobanoglu MA, et al. Serial echocardiographic findings early after heart transplantation: evidence for reversible right ventricular dysfunction and myocardial edema. *J Heart Transplant*. 1987;6:343–7.
15. Kouchoukas NT, Karp RB. Fundamentals of clinical cardiology. *Am Heart J*. 1976;92:513–531.
16. Cohn JN, Franciosa JA: Vasodilator therapy of cardiac failure. *N Engl J Med*. 1977;297:27–31, 254–258.
17. Chatterjee K, Parmley WW. The role of vasodilator therapy in heart failure. *Prog Cardiovasc Dis*. 1977;19:301–325.
18. Sakamoto T, Yamada T. Hemodynamic effects of dobutamine in patients following open heart surgery. *Circulation*. 1977;55:525–533.
19. Fremes SE, Weisel RD, Mickle DG, et al. A comparison of nitroglycerine and nitroprusside: II. The effects of volume loading. *Ann Thorac Surg*. 1985;39:61–67.
20. Lorell B, Leinbach RC, Pohost GM, et al. Right ventricular infarction. *Am J Cardiol*. 1979;43:465–471.

21. Weiss CI, Park JV, Bolman RM: Prostaglandin E_1 for treatment of elevated pulmonary vascular resistance in patients undergoing cardiac transplantation. *Transplant Proc*. 1989;21:2555–2561.
22. Pierce WS, Parr GVS, Myers JL. Ventricular assist pumping in patients with cardiogenic shock after cardiac operation. *N Engl J Med*. 1981;350:1606–1610.
23. Bolooki H. *Clinical Application of the Intra-aortic Balloon Pump*. Mount Kisco, NY: Futura Publishing Co; 1984.
24. Gambert P, Miller JL, Lough ME. Impact of protective isolation on the incidence of infection after heart transplantation. *J Heart Transplant*. 1987;6:147–149.
25. Bennett WM, Norman DJ. Action and toxicity of cyclosporine. *Annu Rev Med*. 1987;37:215–224.

8
Endomyocardial Biopsy: Techniques and Interpretation of Rejection

JUDITH RAY AND JEFFREY D. HOSENPUD

Biopsy of the human heart during life was an uncommon event and performed only during thoracotomy until the early 1950s. Sutton and colleagues[1] first reported percutaneous needle biopsy of the left ventricle in 1956. Bercu et al.[2] developed the technique further and in 1964 reported results from animal and human myocardial biopsies. The earliest experience with the transvascular approach for cardiac biopsy was reported by Sakakibara and Konno in 1962.[3] The cardiac bioptome was a modified cardiac catheter that contained a small jaw at the tip linked by a wire running through the catheter and connected to a moveable handle that could open and close the jaws. Because of its simplicity and relative safety, catheter biopsy of the heart became the technique of choice. Subsequent to the initial report, a variety of minor modifications of the basic technique have been described.[4-9] In 1973 Caves and colleagues first reported the use of transvenous endomyocardial biopsy to diagnose rejection in cardiac allograft recipients.[10] Using a modified bioptome (Fig. 8.1) and the internal jugular vein as vascular access, they were able to perform multiple biopsies on 17 allograft recipients with an overall success rate of 98% and minimal morbidity. Therefore, the concept of using endomyocardial biopsy for rejection surveillance was proven effective in a number of patients in this series.

Currently, the Stanford technique is the most common technique used in the United States. The King's bioptome is a smaller diameter, Teflon-coated modification of the Konno bioptome and is the most commonly used biopsy catheter in Europe. A final major modification of the cardiac biopsy technique is the use of a long sheath placed in the specific chamber to be biopsied. This was originally described by Brooksby and colleagues[12] and has had its major application in left ventricular biopsy and right ventricular biopsy from the femoral vein approach.[8,9]

Survival after cardiac transplantation has steadily improved over the past decade. Although improvement in immunosuppressive agents and overall medical care have played a major role in the increased survival,

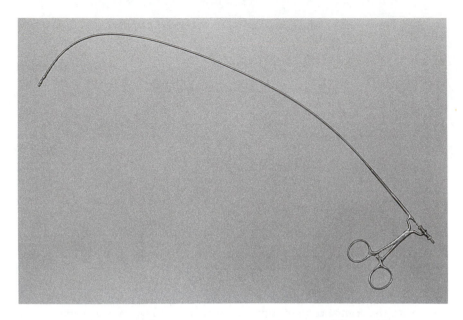

FIGURE 8.1. The Caves-Schulz Bioptome developed at Stanford University. Reproduced from Hosenpud JD.[11] Complications of Endomyocardial Biopsy *In* Kron J, Morton MJ. Complications of Cardiac Catheterization and Angiography: Prevention and Management, 1989, Futura Publishing Co, Inc, Mount Kisco, NY, with permission.

the other major factor has been the use of surveillance endomyocardial biopsies for the diagnosis of rejection. Typically, endomyocardial biopsies are performed weekly for the first month after transplantation; the biopsy frequency is reduced over subsequent months to a baseline frequency of three to four times per year.

Technical Aspects

Right Ventricular Biopsy: Internal Jugular Vein Approach

The usual approach for right ventricular biopsy is through the right internal jugular vein, although the femoral vein has also been used.[3,4,9] The procedure is performed using fluoroscopy. The patient is instructed to take only liquids by mouth for the previous 6 hours. Usually no presedation is required; however, small amounts of a short-acting benzodiazapine can be used. For the right internal jugular approach, the patient is positioned on the fluoroscopy table in the supine position, and the patient's

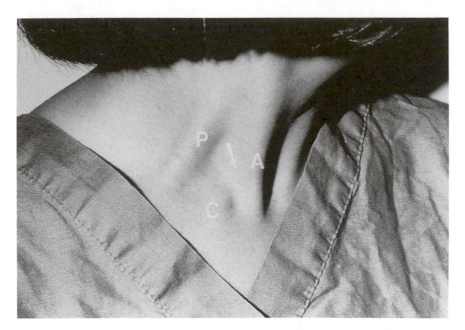

FIGURE 8.2. Landmarks for needle entry into the right internal jugular vein are demonstrated. Note the triangle created by the anterior (A) and posterior (P) heads of the sternocleidomastoid muscle and the clavicle (C). The needle entry point (small arrow) is just lateral to the anterior head, approximately 3 cm. above the clavicle. Reproduced from Hosenpud JD.[11] Complications of Endomyocardial Biopsy *In* Kron J, Morton MJ. Complications of Cardiac Catheterization and Angiography: Prevention and Management, 1989, Futura Publishing Co, Inc, Mount Kisco, NY, with permission.

head is turned completely to the left, bringing both the lateral and medial bellies of the sternocleidomastoid muscle to an anterior position (Fig. 8.2). The legs are raised aproximately 40 cm with soft cushions. The neck is then prepared from chin to approximately 3 cm below the clavicle and draped using sterile technique, exposing the entire triangle bordered by the two bellies of the sternocleidomastoid and the clavicle. The entry site is along the lateral border of the medial belly of the sternocleidomastoid, approximately 2 cm above the clavicle. Local anesthesia is accomplished using 1% lidocaine without epinephrine. Both superficial and deep soft tissue are anesthetized down to but not entering the carotid sheath. Injection of lidocaine into the carotid sheath may tamponade the internal jugular vein, thereby making it difficult to cannulate. The skin is incised approximately 3 mm along the skin lines with a #11 scalpel blade and the subcutaneous tissue is spread with a mosquito clamp. The needle is directed toward the right nipple at an angle of approximately 30° off the

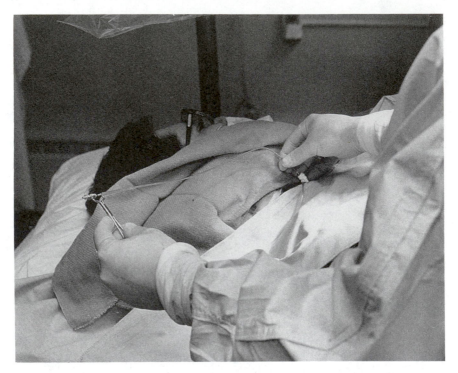

FIGURE 8.3. The bioptome is inserted into the sheath as the patient suspends respiration.

skin. A 20- or 21-gauge 1.5-inch needle may be used to locate the internal jugular vein. The vein is then punctured by an 18-gauge thin-walled needle, through which a 0.035-inch guidewire is passed. The guidewire is advanced into the internal jugular vein to the high right atrium, and its position confirmed by fluoroscopy. A 9 French (F) sheath with side arm, hemostasis valve, and dilator are then advanced over the guidewire, and the guidewire and dilator are removed. The sheath must have a valve at its proximal portion to prevent bleeding through the sheath and embolization of air. The bioptome used at Oregon Health Sciences University is the Caves-Schulz 9F instrument. Before insertion the bioptome is carefully examined to ensure that the jaws approximate tightly and that the 90° bend on the shaft is lined up with the bioptome handle. This enables the operator to know precisely where the bioptome tip is in the vertical (anteroposterior) plane during fluoroscopy.

The side portion of the catheter sheath is flushed with heparinized saline before and between every bioptome insertion. The patient is asked to suspend respiration and the bioptome is inserted (Fig. 8.3). The tip of the catheter is then directed laterally along the superior vena cava and right atrium. One-half to two-thirds of the length down the right atrial

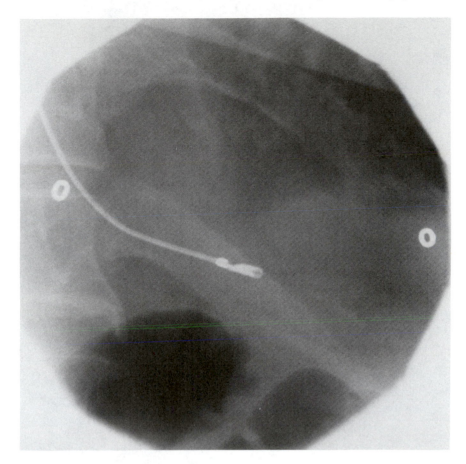

FIGURE 8.4. The bioptome is seen under fluoroscopy with the jaws closed. Reproduced from Hosenpud JD.[11] Complications of Endomyocardial Biopsy *In* Kron J, Morton MJ. Complications of Cardiac Catheterization and Angiography: Prevention and Management, 1989, Futura Publishing Co, Inc, Mount Kisco, NY, with permission.

chamber the bioptome tip is rotated anteriorly across the tricuspid valve and then medially into the right ventricle. As the bioptome is advanced into the right ventricle, the tip is gradually rotated posteriorly so that when the tip approaches the right ventricular apex, it is fully posterior. The tip of the bioptome is then gently abutted against the endocardium (Fig. 8.4), which is appreciated both fluoroscopically and by feeling the cardiac impulse. The tip is then retracted 1 cm, the jaws are opened (Fig. 8.5), the bioptome is advanced again to the endocardial surface, and the jaws are closed. A brisk but gentle tug removes the endomyocardial sample. The bioptome is removed during apnea and the endomyocardial sample is teased gently from the open jaws (Fig. 8.6).

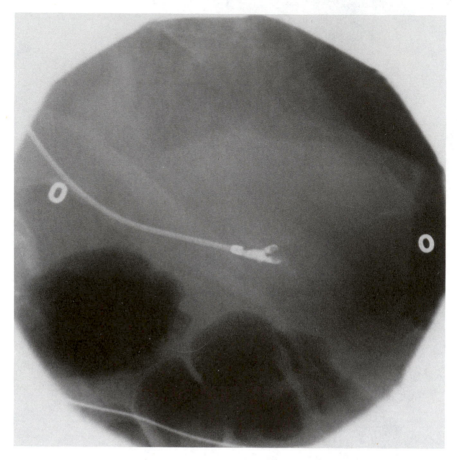

FIGURE 8.5. The bioptome jaws open in preparation for sampling. Reproduced from Hosenpud JD.[11] Complications of Endomyocardial Biopsy *In* Kron J, Morton MJ. Complications of Cardiac Catheterization and Angiography: Prevention and Management, 1989, Futura Publishing Co, Inc, Mount Kisco, NY, with permission.

Right Ventricular Biopsy: Femoral Vein Approach

Although described initially by Sakakibara and Konno[3] and later by Richardson,[4] the femoral vein approach to endomyocardial biopsy is less widely used than venous access from the upper extremities or jugular approaches. More recently, Anderson and Marshall presented a technique for right heart biopsy from the femoral vein using a shaped long-sheath catheter system.[9] They reported using the technique in 35 patients with only one minor complication. The technique used at the Oregon Health Sciences University is a modification of the long-sheath method. The right groin is prepared and draped using sterile technique. Local an-

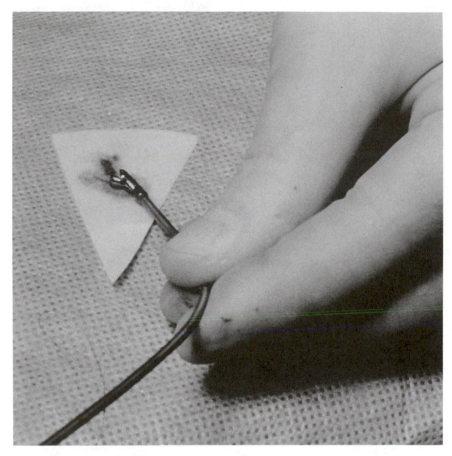

FIGURE 8.6. An endomyocardial sample is gently teased from the open jaws of the bioptome onto a small piece of filter paper. Reproduced from Hosenpud JD.[11] Complications of Endomyocardial Biopsy *In* Kron J, Morton MJ. Complications of Cardiac Catheterization and Angiography: Prevention and Management, 1989, Futura Publishing Co, Inc, Mount Kisco, NY, with permission.

esthesia is accomplished with 1% lidocaine. The entry site for the femoral vein is below the inguinal ligament, just medial to the femoral artery. The skin is opened approximately 3 mm with a #11 scalpel blade and the subcutaneous tissue spread with a blunt clamp. The femoral vein is entered using a thin-wall 18-gauge needle through which a 0.025 inch × 125 cm long Teflon-coated guidewire is inserted and advanced, using fluoroscopy for guidance into the right atrium.

The bioptome used for this technique is a 6F left ventricular biopsy forceps (Cordis Corp., Miami, Fla, and/or Mansfield Scientific Inc., Mansfield, Mass). It is modified by putting a 30° bend 2 cm from the tip. The sheath used is a 6F Mullins sheath/catheter system (USCI Division,

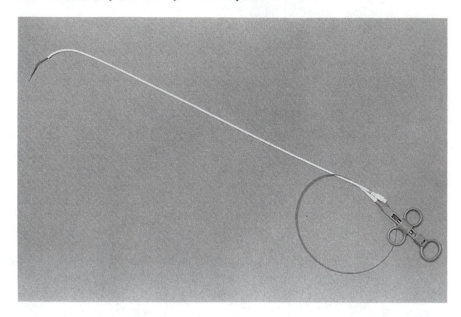

FIGURE 8.7. The bioptome and sheath system used for right ventricular endomyocardial biopsy from the femoral vein. Note the shortened sheath and the bend in the bioptome approximately 2 cm from the tip for anteroposterior positioning (arrows). Reproduced from Hosenpud JD.[11] Complications of Endomyocardial Biopsy *In* Kron J, Morton MJ. Complications of Cardiac Catheterization and Angiography: Prevention and Management, 1989, Futura Publishing Co, Inc, Mount Kisco, NY, with permission.

C.R. Bard Inc., Billerica, Mass), which is also modified by removing a portion of the end of the sheath to convert the 180° curve to 130° to 150°. Fig. 8.7 demonstrates the modified bioptome and sheath system. The sheath and catheter are inserted over the guidewire and advanced into the right atrium. The catheter is manipulated across the tricuspid valve and into the right ventricle with the tip of the sheath just beyond the tricuspid valve annulus. The catheter is removed and the sheath carefully flushed. The bioptome is then inserted through the sheath. As the sheath is just across the tricuspid valve, the bioptome is carefully advanced into the right ventricle. Once the bioptome is advanced near the right ventricular apex it is rotated clockwise, directing the tip posteriorly to ensure that the bioptome is directed toward the interventricular septum. The advantage of not having the sheath positioned more distally is that the bioptome itself can be manipulated to slightly different positions to allow biopsies to be obtained from multiple sites.

We have used this technique successfully on approximately 50 patients with one instance of cardiac perforation on the second patient. The disadvantages of this technique are that it is more time consuming and that the biopsies obtained using this bioptome are substantially smaller (1 mm) and therefore require more samples. For these reasons we use this approach only if the internal jugular vein is not usable.

Left Ventricular Biopsy

Biopsy of the left ventricle should be reserved only for rare instances such as inability to obtain adequate tissue from the right ventricle (multiple prior biopsies) or when the suspicion of rejection is high despite a negative right ventricular biopsy. The only advantage to left ventricular biopsy is the reduced chance for perforation because of the more uniform thickness of the left ventricle. This is far outweighed by the disadvantages of requiring intraarterial access with its potential complications, as well as the concern of systemic arterial embolization. In fact, the need for left ventricular biopsy at Oregon Health Sciences University has been quite limited (one allograft recipient).

The technique is quite similar to routine arterial catheterization. The right or left femoral artery is cannulated with an 18-gauge Seldinger needle and a 0.035-inch $\times$ 125 cm Teflon-coated guidewire is inserted and directed to the diaphragm under fluoroscopy. After dilation of the arteriotomy, a 7F pigtail and sheath combination (Cordis Co., Miami, FL) is inserted over the guidewire and advanced to the abdominal aorta. The wire is removed, the patient is anticoagulated with intravenous heparin (10 units/lb body weight), and the catheter is flushed. The catheter/sheath is then advanced across the aortic valve and into the left ventricle. The pigtail catheter is removed, leaving the sheath in the body of the left ventricle. A Cordis 104-cm. 7F biopsy forceps is then advanced through the sheath into the left ventricle for sampling. The sheath is carefully flushed after each pass of the biopsy forceps to prevent thrombus formation.

Complications of Endomyocardial Biopsy

In general, endomyocardial biopsy in experienced hands is a safe procedure with only rare complications. Based on a large series from Stanford, the overall complication rate is appproximately 1%.[8] Table 8.1 summarizes the complications that are directly referable to the biopsy procedure. Not included are the variety of potential complications associated with arterial cannulation (left ventricular biopsy) because endomyocardial biopsy is performed most often using venous access.

Tissue Processing

Since allograft rejection is a multifocal process, sampling error can contribute to a substantial false-negative rate. For this reason, three to five pieces (depending on bioptome used) of myocardium are necessary for a biopsy to be considered sufficient for evaluation.

TABLE 8.1. Complications of endomyocardial biopsy.

Potential complications	Reported incidence (%)
Cardiac perforation tamponade	0.14
Arrhythmias	0.81
Conduction abnormalities	Rare
Air embolism	0.15
Pneumothorax	0.075
Vascular trauma	Rare
Nerve palsy	
Recurrent laryngeal	0.05
Horner's syndrome	0.025
Overall	1

The pieces of myocardium from biopsy should be fixed immediately in 10% buffered formalin and processed for paraffin embedding. Sections for microscopy are cut 4μ thick at two levels and stained with hematoxylin and eosin and Masson's trichrome. Some institutions also routinely stain sections with methyl green pyronine[13] (to identify RNA synthesis in activated lymphoblasts).

Biopsy Interpretation

Early Graft Injury

Rarely hyperacute rejection involves the transplanted heart. This results from preformed anti-donor human leukocyte antigen antibodies or in cases of ABO incompatibility. The heart turns purple and fibrillates soon after reperfusion. Immediate retransplant is required if the patient is to survive.[14]

The histological changes consist of diffuse interstitial hemorrhage, margination of neutrophils in vessels, and fibrin thrombi and aggregates of erythrocytes blocking capillaries. If the allograft has survived long enough, neutrophils may also be evident in the interstitium of the heart. In general, the changes noted are similar to those seen in acute myocardial infarction, except that the process is diffuse rather than focal.[14] For obvious reasons, the changes of hyperacute rejection are not seen on endomyocardial biopsy but may be noted in an explanted heart or at autopsy.

Interpretation of Endomyocardial Biopsy Ischemic Injury

Ischemic changes in the allograft can be seen during the first week after transplantation and frequently are the most striking changes noted in the

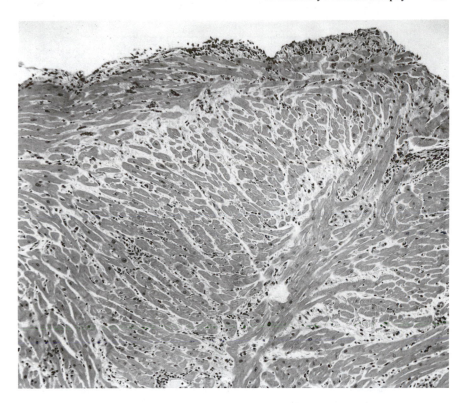

FIGURE 8.8. Endomyocardial biopsy (6 days posttransplantation) showing foci of myocyte damage associated with scant inflammatory infiltrate (hemotoxylin-eosin, × 150; reproduced at 85%).

first allograft biopsy. The earliest recognized histological change of ischemia is a bright, glassy orangeophilia of myocardial fibers with loss of striations and nuclear detail. This is generally not accompanied by an appreciable inflammatory infiltrate (Fig. 8.8). As the lesions progress there is focal loss of myocytes, which may be accompanied by a mild neutrophilic infiltrate.[14] With resolution, histiocytes are noted at the periphery of the ischemic foci followed by a gradual replacement of necrotic myocardium by fibrous connective tissue.

Grading of Acute Rejection

Episodes of acute rejection may occur any time during the life of the allograft, but are most common during the first three months after transplant and are unusual earlier than five days posttransplant.

A number of schemes for characterizing various acute rejection states

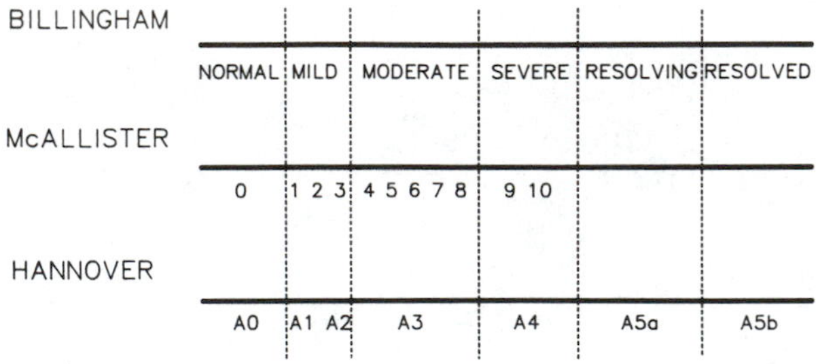

BILLINGHAM

	NORMAL	MILD	MODERATE	SEVERE	RESOLVING	RESOLVED

McALLISTER

	0	1 2 3	4 5 6 7 8	9 10		

HANNOVER

	A0	A1 A2	A3	A4	A5a	A5b

FIGURE 8.9. Three biopsy grading scales currently in use in the United States and Europe. The McAllister scale subdivides all of the categories of rejection into multiple subgroups primarily based on the extent of the myocardium involved. The Hannover method is quite similar to Billingham's criteria.

have been described. Three of these that are recognized and two that are in widespread use will be described (Fig. 8.9).

Billingham's grading system[13,14] includes four categories of acute rejection: mild, moderate, severe, and resolving/resolved.

Mild Acute Rejection

Mild acute rejection is characterized by a sparse perivascular infiltrate of small lymphocytes and lymphoblasts with large nuclei, prominent nucleoli, and pyroninophilic cytoplasm. Interstitial and endocardial edema may be present. Staining with methyl green pyronine may also show pyroninophilia of both endocardial and endothelial cells. Myocyte necrosis is not evident at this stage of rejection, which often reverses spontaneously and is only treated if persistent or progressive (Fig. 8.10).

Moderate Acute Rejection

The next more severe grade of acute rejection is moderate acute rejection. The mononuclear inflammatory infiltrate observed in moderate acute rejection is similar in character but different in degree and location from that seen in mild acute rejection. The early changes of moderate acute rejection include increased density of perivascular inflammation and extension of the infiltrate into the interstitium, with lymphoblasts separating groups of myocytes and surrounding individual myocardial fibers (Fig. 8.11). Plasma cells may also be a more prominent component. Later in the course of moderate acute rejection, foci of inflammation are larger and more numerous. Focal myocyte necrosis is often identified in myocardium adjacent to an inflammatory focus. This is characterized on hematoxylin and eosin-stained sections by shrunken, pale, often fragmented myocytes. Individual myofibers may appear to be invaded by the inflammatory infiltrate. Necrosis is frequently more evident on trichrome-stained sections where necrotic myocytes appear shrunken and

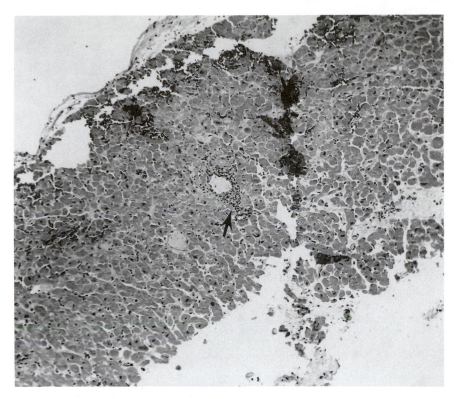

FIGURE 8.10. Endomyocardial biopsy showing the slight perivascular mononuclear infiltration (arrow) of mild acute rejection (hemotoxylin-eosin, × 150; reproduced at 85%).

gray in contrast to the eosinophilia of normal myocardial cells. The changes of moderate acute rejection, both early and late, are considered reversible with appropriate therapy.

Severe Acute Rejection

Severe acute rejection is rarely seen and is considered difficult or impossible to reverse. Inflammation is more intense and widespread and the inflammatory infiltrate frequently includes eosinophils and neutrophils. Myocyte necrosis is readily identified and may involve large confluent areas of myocardium. Interstitial hemorrhage associated with damaged vessels and microthrombi is also frequently present.

A diagnosis of acute rejection of any degree will prompt rebiopsy usually within 2 weeks. Histological evaluation of the follow-up biopsy is done in conjunction with the previous biopsy. If the changes noted are the same or worse than previously seen, the acute rejection is said to be ongoing.

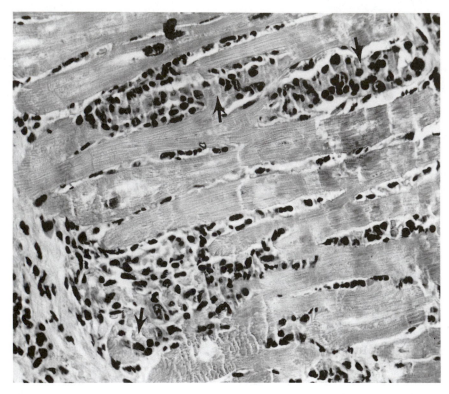

FIGURE 8.11. Endomyocardial biopsy showing moderate acute rejection with interstitial inflammation. Arrows delineate areas of myocyte necrosis (hemotoxylin-eosin, × 675; reproduced at 85%).

Resolving/Resolved

Treatment of an acute rejection episode often results in reduction of the inflammatory infiltrate within 36 to 72 hours. Follow-up biopsy then reveals reduced numbers of mononuclear cells and may show fibroblasts indicative of early scar formation. These changes warrant the diagnosis of resolving rejection. Myocyte necrosis after ischemia or acute rejection resolves more slowly so that even though inflammation may largely subside in a matter of days, necrotic myocytes may persist for 2 or more weeks. Persistent myocyte necrosis in the presence of declining inflammation should not be interpreted as ongoing acute rejection.[14,15]

A rejection episode is "resolved" 1 to 2 weeks after therapy for acute rejection when scar replaces the areas of inflammation and necrosis. Residual mononuclear cells may be present but are nonpyroninophilic and frequently are "trapped" in the scar, where they may persist for many weeks (Fig. 8.12).

The grading system of acute rejection developed by McAllister and col-

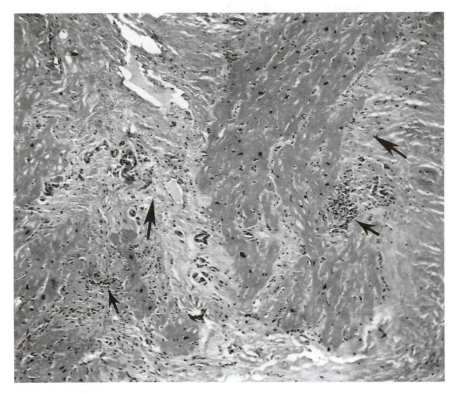

FIGURE 8.12. Biopsy of scarred myocardium (large arrows) with "trapped" lymphocytes (smaller arrows) (hemotoxylin-eosin, × 150; reproduced at 85%).

leagues[16] at the Texas Heart Institute is similar to that of the Stanford group. This scheme divides acute rejection on a scale from 0 to 10. A value of 0 is given if there is no evidence of rejection. A grade of 1 or 2 is applied to those biopsies showing perivascular aggregates of mononuclear cells and corresponds to Billingham's "mild acute rejection". Grade 3 represents perivascular inflammation and infiltration of mononuclear cells into interstitium without myocyte degeneration. Grades 4 to 8 correspond to "moderate acute rejection" of the Stanford grading system. In grade 4 interstitial inflammation is present, as are rare small foci of myocyte necrosis. With increasing severity of rejection foci of inflammation become more numerous, intensity of inflammation increases, and myocyte necrosis becomes more obvious. These changes are reflected in progressively higher grades of rejection. Grade 8, therefore, shows multifocal myocyte necrosis with associated intense mononuclear inflammation. Grades 9 and 10 show extensive myocyte degeneration, interstitial hemorrhage, and a mixed interstitial inflammatory infiltrate, including polymorphonuclear leukocytes, and corresponds to severe rejection in Billingham's scheme.

A modification of Billingham's classification, of rejection is the Hannover classification, which has gained popularity in Europe. It grades acute rejection on a scale of A0 to A4 (no rejection to severe rejection) with A-5a and A-5b being resolving and resolved respectively, chronic rejection C-0 or C-1 (absent or present), vasculopathy B-0 to B-2 (none to severe), fibrosis F-0 or F-1 (absent or present), and nonrejection related changes E-0 or E-1 (absent or present).[17]

Difficulties Encountered in Biopsy Interpretation

Several problems may be encountered that confound the accurate diagnosis of acute rejection in an allograft biopsy.

The first of these is ischemic myocardial injury, which has been previously discussed.[18] In ischemic change myocyte necrosis may be quite prominent and may be accompanied by an acute inflammatory infiltrate. Of help in differentiating ischemia from acute rejection (which may also be present) is the paucity of inflammation in relation to the amount of necrosis in ischemic injury, as opposed to more intense mononuclear infiltration in acute rejection accompanied by little or no myocyte damage[14] (Fig. 8.8).

Another difficulty of interpretation arises with cyclosporine "Quilty" phenomenon.[14] This is an inflammatory infiltrate of pyroninophilic T lymphocytes present focally in the endocardium. Difficulty with distinguishing this effect from acute rejection is encountered when the infiltrate extends for some distance into myocardium and overlying endocardium becomes detached or is not recognized (Fig. 8.13).

The inflammatory infiltrate accompanying an infectious agent may be confused with the infiltrate of acute rejection. However, inflammation generally associated with microorganisms is a mixed inflammatory infiltrate in contrast to the mononuclear cell infiltrate of rejection.[14]

Previous endomyocardial biopsy sites can be confused with acute allograft rejection.[14,18] Because patients are biopsied frequently and the same area of right ventricle is sampled each time, it is common to biopsy a site previously biopsied. If the biopsy site is a recent one the endocardium will be disrupted and replaced by a cap of fibrin and inflammatory cells with subjacent granulation tissue (Fig. 8.14). Older biopsy sites show varying amounts of collagen with evidence of old hemorrhage and myofiber disarray (Fig. 8.15).

Changes Attributed to Cyclosporine

Some changes noted in endomyocardial biopsies are peculiar to cyclosporine-treated patients.[14] The most striking of these is "Quilty ef-

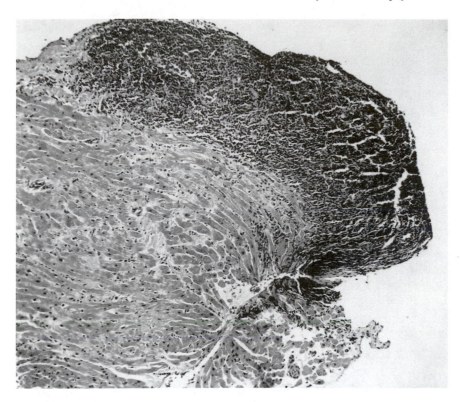

FIGURE 8.13. Endomyocardial biopsy showing cyclosporine "Quilty" phenomenon described as a subendocardial, well demarcated lymphocytic infiltrate. In this example there is some extension of inflammatory infiltrate into myocardial interstitium (hemotoxylin-eosin, × 150; reproduced at 85%).

fect'', which consists of focal endocardial lymphocytic infiltrates. This phenomenon is not understood, but occurs only in cyclosporine-treated patients and does not require treatment unless acute rejection is identified elsewhere in the biopsy.

Eosinophils that are rarely seen in conventionally treated patients except in the presence of myocardial infection are a fairly common component of moderate and severe acute rejections in cyclosporine treated patients.[14]

Fibrosis from healed rejection episodes, ischemia, or prior endomyocardial biopsies is present in all cardiac allografts,[14] but fine patchy perimyocyte fibrosis is characteristic of cyclosporine treatment and is apparently dose-dependent.[14]

Cyclosporine-treated patients are slower to develop rejection episodes.[14] Five to 7 days are generally required to develop moderate acute rejection after a mild acute rejection episode in a cyclosporine-treated

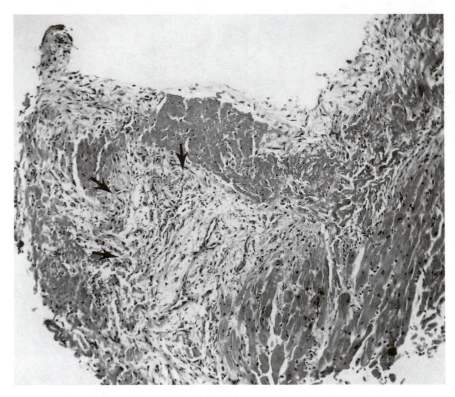

FIGURE 8.14. Recent biopsy site with fibrin cap and underlying granulation tissue (arrows) (hemotoxylin-eosin, × 150; reproduced at 85%).

patient, whereas it may develop in only 48 hours in an azathioprine-treated patient. Similarly, resolution of acute rejection is much slower in cyclosporine-treated patients—moderate acute rejection frequently takes one to two weeks to resolve.[14]

Infectious Agents

Infection is the most frequent cause of death in cardiac transplant patients.[14] Usually the infection is systemic and may involve any number of pathogenic or opportunistic microorganisms. Occasionally, microorganisms are noted on routine endomyocardial biopsy. Those most commonly encountered are *Toxoplasma gondii* and cytomegalovirus. The presence of an inflammatory infiltrate, including eosinophils (even in cyclosporine-treated patients), should prompt a careful examination of all sectioned tissue fragments for organisms. Cytomegalovirus or cysts of toxoplasma may, on occasion, fail to elicit an inflammatory response (Fig. 8.16).

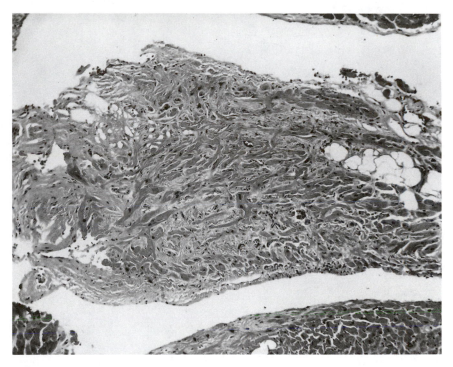

FIGURE 8.15. Healed endomyocardial biopsy site showing myocyte disarray and fibrosis (hemotoxylin-eosin, × 150; reproduced at 85%).

Chronic Rejection

Among the most significant reasons for late allograft loss is chronic rejection. Some of the changes observed in chronic rejection may be noted on endomyocardial biopsy, but usually are more evident in the explanted heart.

Chronic rejection, as evidenced by the striking changes noted in the coronary arteries and small vessels of the myocardium, is presumed to be the result of previous repeated episodes of immunological damage to the intima followed by reparative myointimal proliferation in a manner similar to that seen in naturally occurring atherosclerosis.[14,18,19]

In chronic rejection the heart is grossly enlarged and coronary arteries and their epicardial branches show thickened walls with lumina narrowed by yellow lipid deposits with or without superimposed thrombus.[20] The myocardium may show areas of fibrosis, but changes of acute infarction are unusual.

Microscopically, the heart may show any or all of the features of acute rejection[14,20] (i.e., edema, perivascular or interstitial inflammation, and myocyte necrosis) or may be without any evidence of acute rejection.

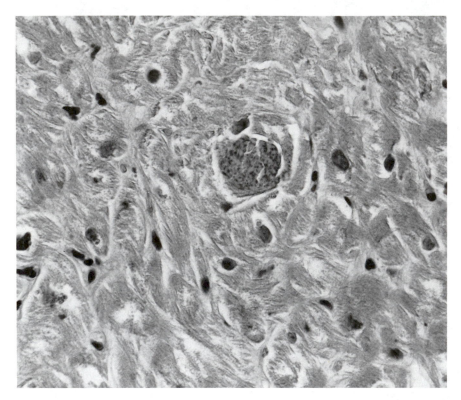

FIGURE 8.16. Cyst of *Toxoplasma gondii* found on routine endomyocardial biopsy. Note absence of inflammatory response (hemotoxylin-eosin, × 885; reproduced at 85%).

The coronary arteries are narrowed by concentric intimal proliferation extending along the length of the vessel and into small epicardial and intramyocardial branches. The intimal lesion is composed of lipid-laden macrophages and modified smooth muscle cells[14,20] (Fig. 8.17). The lesions rarely disrupt the internal elastic lamina and rarely calcify. These changes are in contrast to those of naturally occurring atherosclerosis in which the lesions are asymmetric and focal and not infrequently calcify.[14]

The lesions of chronic rejection, like those of naturally occurring atherosclerosis, can lead to myocardial ischemia and frequently result in graft failure.

Conclusion

The surveillance endomyocardial biopsy has been a major advance in the management of patients after cardiac transplantation. It is a safe procedure from multiple approaches in experienced hands. Care must be taken

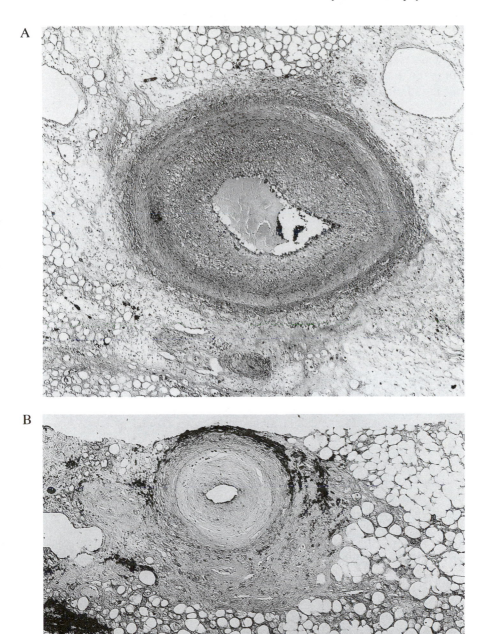

FIGURE 8.17. A, Concentric intimal proliferation of chronic rejection in coronary artery and B, Epicardial branch in cardiac allograft of 20 months' duration (hemotoxyin-eosin, × 58 and × 67, respectively; reproduced at 85% and 70%, respectively).

to obtain adequate tissue for interpretation, especially in patients who have undergone multiple biopsies. Finally, the interpretation of the biopsy material requires substantial expertise not only in cardiac pathology but in the diagnosis and follow-up of allograft rejection to avoid the potential pitfalls in biopsy interpretation.

References

1. Sutton DC, Sutton GC, Kent G. Needle biopsy of the human ventricular myocardium. *Bull Northwest Univ Med Sch*. 1956;30:213–221.
2. Bercu B, Heinz J, Choudhry AS, Cabrera P. Myocardial biopsy: a new technique utilizing the ventricular septum. *Am J Cardiol*. 1964;14:675–678.
3. Sakakibara S, Konno S. Endomyocardial biopsy. *Jpn Heart J*. 1962;3:537–542.
4. Richardson PJ. King's endomyocardial bioptome. *Lancet*. 1974;1:660–661.
5. Caves PK, Schulz WP, Dong E Jr, Stinson EB, Shumway NE. New instrument for transvenous cardiac biopsy. *Am J Cardiol*. 1974;33:264–267.
6. Ali N. Transvenous endomyocardial biopsy using the gastrointestinal biopsy (Olympus GFB) catheter. *Am Heart J*. 1974;87:294–297.
7. Lurie PR, Fujita M, Neustein HB. Transvascular endomyocardial biopsy in infants and small children: description of a new technique. *Am J Cardiol*. 1978;42:453–457.
8. Mason JW. Techniques for right and left ventricular endomyocardial biopsy. *Am J Cardiol*. 1978;41:887–892.
9. Anderson JL, Marshall HW. The femoral venous approach to endomyocardial biopsy: comparison with internal jugular and transarterial approaches. *Am J Cardiol*. 1984;53:833–837.
10. Caves PK, Stinson EB, Billingham M, Shumway NE. Percutaneous transvenous endomyocardial biopsy in human heart recipients. Experience with a new technique. *Ann Thorac Surg*. 1973;16:325–336.
11. Hosenpud JD. Complications of endomyocardial biopsy. In: Kron J, Morton MJ, eds. *Complications of Cardiac Catheterization and Angiography: Prevention and Management*. Mt. Kisco, NY: Futura Publishing Co; 1989.
12. Brooksby IAB, Swanton RH, Jenkins BS, Webb-Peploe MM. Long-sheath technique for introduction of catheter tip manometer or endomyocardial bioptome into left or right heart. *Br Heart J*. 1974;36:908–912.
13. Billingham ME. Diagnosis of cardiac rejection by endomyocardial biopsy. *J Heart Transplant*. 1981;1:25–30.
14. Billingham ME. The postsurgical heart. *Am J Cardiovasc Pathol*. 1988:1:319–334.
15. Carrier M, Paplonus SH, Graham AR, Copeland JG. Histopathology of acute myocardial necrosis: effects of immunosuppression therapy. *J Heart Transplant*. 1987:6:218–221.
16. McAllister HA Jr, Schnee MJM, Radovancevic B, Frazier OH. A system for grading cardiac allograft rejection. *Texas Heart Inst J*. 1986:13:1–3.
17. Kemnitz J, Cohnert T, Schafers HJ, Helmke M, et al. A classification of cardiac allograft rejection. *Am J Surg Pathol*. 1987:11:503–515.

18. Pomerance A, Stovin PGI. Heart transplant pathology: the British experience. *J Clin Pathol.* 1985:38:146–159.
19. Uys CJ, Rose AG. Pathologic findings in long term cardiac transplants. *Arch Path Lab Med.* 1984:108:112–116.
20. Uys CJ, Rose AG. The pathology of cardiac transplantation. In: Silver, M, ed. *Cardiovascular Pathology.* New York, NY: Churchill Livingstone; 1983:1329–1352.

9
Chronic Immunosuppression and the Treatment of Acute Rejection

DANIEL R. SALOMON AND MARIAN C. LIMACHER

The proper management of immunosuppression in cardiac transplantation requires a working knowledge of immunology and pharmacology. In practice, most centers now employ two to four different immunosuppressive drugs in one of several complicated protocols. If one considers the considerable variability of individual patients, the potential for multiple drug interactions, and the significant compliance problems inherent in any chronic multidrug regimen, then the dimensions of the challenge immunosuppression represents to the practicing physician becomes apparent. Therefore, this chapter will review each of the drugs now used for immunosuppression (Fig. 9.1), describe most of the multidrug protocols currently in use, and evaluate the drug side effects and potential interactions.

The Challenge of Immunosuppression in Practice

If an immunosuppressive protocol is inadequate the patient may develop acute or chronic rejection that threatens his graft survival or his life. On the other hand, if the patient is over-immunosuppressed, the risk of lethal infection or malignancy is very real. Whereas these two basic tenets of practice are intellectually straightforward, the act of balancing these problems in clinical practice is not.

First, the transplant physician should never follow an immunosuppressive protocol rigidly despite the fact that conformity is often reassuring. Immunosuppression must be individualized like any drug therapy and it must change in response to the changes in the patient's clinical course. For example, if a patient has a major surgical complication and for any of numerous reasons becomes malnourished or debilitated, one might reduce the immunosuppression, particularly the steroids, to protect the patient from infection and promote wound healing. Note that it is often necessary to decrease the immunosuppression judiciously during acute infections, most commonly with cytomegalovirus (CMV). It remains the

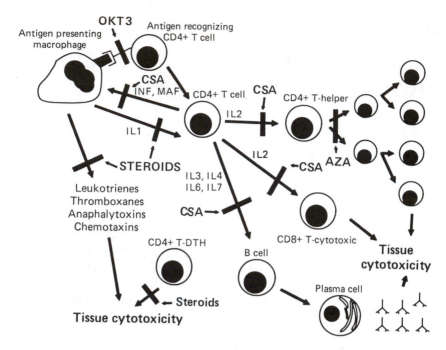

FIGURE 9.1. A schematic representation of the immune response and the effects of the commonly used immunosuppressive agents *(see text)*. CSA = cyclosporine, AZA = azathioprine, IL-1–7 = interleukins 1–7, INF = gamma interferon, MAF = macrophage activating factor.

art of transplantation to determine when this should be undertaken and when the immunosuppression can be safely increased again.

Second, the typical focus of our attention in the first few months after transplantation is rejection and the frequent clinic visits are centered on numerous endomyocardial biopsies. As a consequence, there is a built-in anxiety to treat rejection whenever diagnosed. In our experience, many episodes of mild and even moderate rejection resolve spontaneously with time or simple enhancements in the immunosuppression, such as by increasing the cyclosporine level or the dose of azathioprine. The transplant physician should review the endomyocardial biopsies with the pathologist and use the trends demonstrated with serial biopsies to evaluate and direct therapy. A more conservative approach to aggressive antirejection therapy will significantly reduce the overall immunosuppression used in a transplant program to the overall benefit of all the patients.

Finally, one must consider long-term care that often threatens to become increasingly routine as patient visit intervals stretch to months and the more acute demands of new patients command our attention. The practice of tapering the immunosuppression in the first months reinforces a tendency to taper the drugs or at least allow cyclosporine levels to fall well below those demanded earlier as long as the most recent biopsy is negative. Nonetheless, it has become evident that accelerated atherosclerosis, which most believe is a form of chronic rejection, is very common and threatens long-term patient and graft survival.[1-5] In fact, this theme is also being recognized in renal transplantation in which long-term renal graft survival in the cyclosporine era has not changed in the same dramatic fashion that short-term survival has improved.[6] Therefore, the careful maintenance of adequate immunosuppression in all patients (especially in those clinically stable) may be extremely important to long-term survival. Reducing the azathioprine dose in a patient at 2 years to improve the hematocrit, reducing the cyclosporine dose to improve blood pressure control, or reducing steroids to decrease lipoprotein levels may all be positive medical maneuvers but inappropriate for immunosuppression. Rather, we must always pay careful attention to cyclosporine levels, continue education and reinforcement of compliance, and, finally, accept the fact that transplantation demands a price of all patients that time does not excuse.

Individual Immunosuppressive Drugs

Azathioprine

History

Azathioprine was first recognized in 1959 via one of its primary metabolites, 6-mercaptopurine, which was reported to inhibit the response of rabbits to immunization with foreign proteins.[7] The exciting possibility that this immunosuppressive effect could be used in transplantation was demonstrated in dogs by Calne in 1960[8] and in 1975 the nitroimidazole derivative, azathioprine, was synthesized and shown to be somewhat less toxic.[9,10] In the next 2 years clinical application in renal transplantation clearly demonstrated the therapeutic value of this drug.[11-14]

Mechanisms

Azathioprine is metabolized by the liver into 6-mercaptopurine as well as a number of metabolites expressing several different mechanisms of immunosuppression.[10] Both deoxyribonucleic acid (DNA) and ribonucleic acid (RNA) synthesis can be inhibited, de novo purine synthesis is blocked, and breaks in the chromosomal DNA may be created.[15,16] Overall, the effect of azathioprine is best understood as an inhibition of cell proliferation. Because cell proliferation initiated by the immune response to foreign antigen is a major step in expanding the T- and B-cell clones that mediate the effector phase of rejection, the role of azathioprine is a potent but nonspecific suppression.

Clinical Use

Azathioprine's immunosuppression is roughly correlated with its major side effect of marrow suppression and most typically represents a lowered leukocyte count. Therefore, in practice most protocols start therapy with a dose of 1.5 to 2 mg/kg, and closely follow the patient's leukocyte count, aiming for a baseline of 5 to 8 $\times$ 10^3 cells/mm^3. It is important to remember that prednisone at high doses will elevate the leukocyte count, especially in the perioperative period, to levels as high as 20 to 25 $\times$ 10^3 because of demargination. Therefore, decisions regarding the ultimate dosage of azathioprine should be deferred until the prednisone dose has been reduced to lower levels (30–40 mg/day). In fact, changes in patient weight and time after transplantation may dictate changes in the dose even a year posttransplantation. Azathioprine may also cause a significant anemia (Hct <30%) and adjustment of the dose in individual patients may be required. There is some controversy surrounding the extent of the linkage between total blood counts and the immunosuppressive effects of azathioprine. One must consider that the immunosuppression of this drug may be reflected by the effect on the blood counts and, therefore, preventing rejection must be balanced against the minimal clinical significance of a mild anemia. Rarely, azathioprine may cause a pure red cell aplasia[17] or profound thrombocytopenia.[18] In these cases the drug should be discontinued or the dose reduced significantly. The common use of sulfamethoxazole/trimethoprim (Septra or Bactrim DS 1 qHS) for the prophylaxis of pneumocystis pneumonia may increase the incidence of thrombocytopenia with azathioprine and, thus, an alternative is to stop the sulfa drug. If this occurs early posttransplant (i.e., <6 months) the same degree of pneumocystis protection can be obtained with pentamidine inhaled once each month. Because the enzyme xanthine oxidase is essential in controlling levels of 6–mercaptopurine (a major metabolite of azathioprine), concomitant use of allopurinol requires that the dose of azathioprine be reduced approximately 75% to avoid toxicity related to excessive immunosuppression and hematologic abnormalities.[15]

Complications

Azathioprine complications include an increased risk of malignancy, particularly skin cancers.[19] Every transplant patient should be carefully advised about limiting sun exposure and the proper selection and use of sun-blocking agents. Careful physical exams at all clinic visits and early biopsy of any suspicious skin lesions are critical. In addition, the general increase in malignancy with this drug suggests increased attention to symptoms of bowel dysfunction, melena, hematuria, and uterine or vaginal bleeding.[19–21] More benign complications such as warts and cutaneous fungal infections are also seen frequently. Azathioprine has been reported to cause liver disease and even failure,[22] though these are case reports and very uncommon. Pancreatitis has also been associated with this drug in patients with inflammatory bowel disease,[23] though its significance in patients with chronic inflammatory diseases and transplant patients is unknown.

Corticosteroids

History

Although the metabolic importance of a crude steroid preparation called Cortin was recognized as early as 1927 in adrenalectomized cats,[24] the value of steroids in immunosuppression evolved more by luck and clinical experience than scientific revelation. Adrenocorticotrophic hormone (ACTH) was purified in 1943,[25,26] chemically identified in 1956,[27] and not synthesized until 1963.[28] In the late 1950s the clinical similarity of renal failure and adrenal failure (hypothermia, hyponatremia, malaise, weakness, pallor, etc.), combined with the pioneering work of George Thorn in Boston with ACTH, led to the empiric use of ACTH in low doses in the first renal transplants done at the Peter Bent Brigham hospital.[29] John Merrill noted the temporal relationship of an ACTH bolus to a temporary improvement in the function of an acutely rejecting renal graft. Within a year the use of prednisone became standard protocol at a number of transplant centers.[13,14,30]

Mechanisms

Steroids in transplantation refer to the intravenous preparation of methyl-prednisolone (Solu-Medrol) and the oral preparations of prednisone or prednisolone (Medrol). Steroids have several mechanisms of action. They inhibit the antigen-presenting macrophages from releasing soluble factors or the cytokines, interleukin-1 (IL-1)[31] and IL-6.[32] These are very important because IL-1 is one of the first signals to activated T cells resulting in the expression of their IL-2 receptors[33] and in some situations IL-6 may supply a necessary coordinate signal.[34] Without an IL-2 receptor the T cells will not proliferate.[35] The steroids also work via a form of feedback inhibition because normally the IL-2 activated T cells would also secrete the lymphokine gamma interferon, and this lymphokine enhances the macrophage's release of more IL-1 and IL-6.[36]

IL-1 is also called endogenous pyrogen[31] and, thus, the inhibition of IL-1 release by steroids explains why patients will promptly lyse their fevers and also be less likely to mount a fever in response to a potentially serious infection. Because the endogenous pyrogen effect of IL-1 is mediated via the hypothalamus, this lymphokine represents one link between the immune response and the central nervous system.

The cellular mechanism of steroids in both macrophages and T cells involves the inhibition of gene transcription for the cytokines described.

Steroids cross the cell membrane, are bound to intracytoplasmic steroid binding molecules, and are transported across the nuclear membrane to bind specific sites located near the cytokine genes and their machinery for transcription and regulation.[37] These sites are called glucocorticoid response elements (GRE) and binding of the steroid/protein complex results in the inhibition of gene transcription.[38] If no messenger RNA is synthesized by transcription of the proper genes then no cytokine can be made by the protein synthetic machinery of the cells. This growing understanding of the molecular basis for steroid action may lead to alternative strategies for blocking cytokine gene transcription that avoid the many nonspecific steroid side effects that will be described below.

The other immunosuppressive mechanism of steroids is their potent antiinflammatory effect. Steroids inhibit macrophage release of inflammatory mediators, such as the leukotrienes, thromboxanes, and anaphalytoxins[39], the release of various chemotaxins necessary for the influx of neutrophils[39], and the delayed-type hypersensitivity cells that may mediate cytotoxicity to local tissues.[40] Thus, it must be remembered that rejection is only initiated by an antigen specific immune response triggered by the foreign antigen of the transplanted organ. However, once rejection begins, the antigen nonspecific cascade of lymphokine release, complement and clotting factor activation, and inflammatory mediators (such as thromboxane) all create a site of acute inflammatory injury that plays a major role in graft damage. Therefore, even if the immunosuppression fails to prevent a rejection episode the antiinflammatory benefits of steroids remain extremely important to protecting the transplanted heart.

Clinical Use

Although the basic strategy is the same, there is great variation between individual centers in their steroid dose protocols. In general, most centers administer 0.5 to 1.5 gm of methylprednisolone intravenously on the first day, during and immediately after surgery. Thereafter, an initial dose of prednisone ranging from 1 to 2.5 mg/kg is given daily and the dose tapered progressively over time. Most programs aim for a baseline prednisone dose of 10 mg/day by the third or fourth month posttransplant (the different protocols will be discussed in the next section). Older patients, children, and diabetic patients should have their steroid doses tapered more aggressively. Ultimate conversion to alternate-day steroid regimens has been attempted in renal transplantation and although a reduction in some steroid side effects has been documented,[41-43] this approach to therapy has not been generally accepted. Furthermore, the value in heart transplantation remains unknown.

Complications

Steroid side effects may be divided as short- and long-term. In the short term it is frequent to see significant mood alterations, sleep disorders, exaggerated anxiety, acne, hirsutism, rapid weight gains, fluid retention with edema, and the classic truncal obesity with a "moon" facies.[44,45] The steroid acne is seen in almost all patients as a diffuse, erythematous, pustular eruption concentrated over the back, chest, and forehead. Topical antibiotics, soaps, and dessicants are usually not successful; however, in most patients the acne will resolve within 6 months as the steroid dose is reduced. The sleep alterations respond poorly to sedatives and these drugs usually exacerbate the mood alterations that are common. Symptoms of gastric irritation and reflux are common and respond well to H2 blockers. Many centers place patients on ranitidine (150 mg BID) immediately postoperatively and discontinue the drug when the steroid dose is reduced to maintenance levels.

Hypertension occurs in most heart transplant patients and the cause is multifactorial. However, in the reported experience with protocols for stopping or avoiding steroids it is clear that the incidence and degree of hypertension is improved.[46] This is also true in the renal transplant literature.[47] In the long term the steroids cause elevations of cholesterol and triglycerides[48–50] even if the original disease of the patient was an idiopathic cardiomyopathy. Obesity remains a major and frustrating problem and this impacts negatively on hypertension management, rehabilitation, and lipoprotein abnormalities. Dietary control and regular exercise remain the most valuable therapies, but as many as one-third of patients will require drug therapy of the lipoprotein abnormalities. Finally, steroid bone disease, including aseptic necrosis and osteoporosis, must be considered.[45]

Cyclosporine

History

Cyclosporine has clearly been responsible for making heart transplantation an effective therapy in end-stage cardiac disease. Cyclosporine was first studied as an antifungal agent in 1972 after its isolation from two species of yeast by Jean Borel.[51,52] Although the drug "failed" evaluation as an antifungal drug because it potently inhibited cellular immune responses in the standard testing, it was fortunate that Borel recognized its potential as an immunosuppressive drug.[52,53] After a series of successful animal transplant experiments[54–56] and trials in Europe with kidney transplantation,[57–61] it was introduced in the early 1980s for heart transplantation. Survival rates in heart transplantation rapidly rose into the 75% to 80% range at 1 year.[62] The success of this drug for immunosuppression, coupled with improved organ procurement and preservation as well as a growing experience with the endomyocardial biopsy, resulted in an explosive growth of successful heart transplant programs between 1982 and 1988.[63]

Mechanisms

Cyclosporine is a T cell-specific drug and it results in potent inhibition of T-cell lymphokine production.[64,65] Almost all the known lymphokines including gamma interferon and IL-2 through IL-7 are potently inhibited by the presence of cyclosporine.[65,66] Note that cyclosporine has no direct inhibitory effect on macrophage production of IL-1[67] but may ultimately reduce IL-1 production by inhibiting T-cell release of gamma interferon. Thus, cyclosporine uses the same feedback inhibition loop as steroids but acts via a different cell and lymphokine. Therefore, cyclosporine and steroids are actually synergistic in their effects on the immune response, which is the basic rationale behind their combined use in transplantation.

The effect of inhibiting lymphokine production on the immune response is profound. Lymphokines represent one of the primary signalling mechanisms in the sequential activation and proliferation of immune T and B cells both for killing (e.g., cell-mediated cytotoxicity) and the production of antibody (e.g., humoral-mediated immunity).[68] The classic example is the lymphokine IL-2, which is produced by activated T helper cells (CD4 positive) after they have been exposed to foreign antigen by the antigen-presenting cells or macrophages.[69] IL-2 is a powerful signal for T-cell proliferation and the expression of IL-2 receptors on the surface of other antigen-activated T cells is the key first step in expanding the clones of killer T cells that will traffic back to the transplant and cause rejection.[70] On the other hand, the inhibition of other T-cell lymphokines such as IL-3, IL-4, IL-6, and IL-7 may result in significant inhibition of B-cell differentiation and proliferation.[71] Therefore, the effect of cyclosporine is to inhibit both the cellular and humoral limbs of the immune response.

The precise mechanism of cyclosporine's inhibition of lymphokine production remains unclear. Cyclosporine inhibits lymphokine gene transcription[72] and, thus, messenger RNA for these lymphokines is not available for the cell's protein machinery. Cyclosporine may interact with the regulatory regions of the genes in much the same manner as the steroids. For example, a specific drug-binding protein for cyclosporine has been identified in both the cytoplasm and nucleus of T cells called cyclophilin.[73] Crabtree and colleagues have recently published evidence of a complex multiple-gene interaction pathway resulting in inhibition of IL-2 gene transcription[74] Cyclophilin has also been shown to be a member of an enzyme family located in the cytoplasm called peptidyl-prolyl cis-trans isomerases,[75] which are important in normal protein folding during protein synthesis. When cyclosporine binds the cyclophilin the enzyme loses its activity. Therefore, cyclosporine may have its effect on some type of cytoplasmic protein-based signal that is required to initiate normal lymphokine gene transcription in the nucleus. All of this is especially interesting when we realize that the new immunosuppressive drug, FK 506, also binds a unique cytoplasmic protein that turns out to be a member of the same enzyme family of proline isomerases (see below).

Clinical Use

In most instances, patients receive an oral loading dose of cyclosporine of between 8 and 15 mg/kg preoperatively on the night before surgery, followed by 8 to 10 mg/kg per day divided into two doses. Most patients can tolerate the oral doses within a few hours after the transplant surgery. However, some centers use intravenous cyclosporine ($\frac{1}{3}$ the oral dose) in the early postoperative period. When given orally, these daily doses are timed after breakfast and dinner so that the routine of taking cyclosporine with meals is well established before discharge. Cyclosporine levels are measured frequently and the dose is adjusted to coincide with target levels for immunosuppression (see below).

Cyclosporine is a difficult drug to use in clinical practice because of the tremendous variability in the dose/level relationship.[76,77] First, cyclosporine is a highly lipophilic drug,[78] which means that its absorption is altered by the fat content of meals and the release of bile acids into the proximal jejunum. Alterations in gastrointestinal function resulting from previous surgery, diabetic enteropathy, ileus, malabsorption, or viral gastroenteritis may profoundly decrease cyclosporine drug absorption, which at best is about 30% of the oral dose.[76] This is a major cause of the significant patient-to-patient variability in the dose required to achieve or maintain a given target level. Second, cyclosporine metabolism changes as a function of time after transplantation such that a progressively lower dose is required over the first 3 months to obtain the same baseline cyclosporine levels.[79] Therefore, levels must be followed very frequently and dose changes made as often as weekly. Third, cyclosporine is subject to many major drug interactions that may cause the drug to go from toxic to subtherapeutic ranges in a few days (see Table 9.1). Given the central importance of cyclosporine to successful transplantation, the transplant physician must accept the burden of following the levels literally forever and actively encouraging patient education and compliance at every opportunity.

Practical Guidelines for Dose Changes

Cyclosporine dose changes must follow several guidelines. First, in routine practice the dose should not be changed more than 20% at any single time. The new steady state level after a dose change will take 10 to 21 days to be reached, although a significant change can be seen in 5 to 10 days. Therefore, if frequent levels are obtained and doses are changed frequently (i.e., every 3 to 7 days), the final level will not be reflected for 3 weeks after the last dose alteration. Second, if a patient with a stable

TABLE 9.1. Cyclosporine drug interactions.

Drugs that lower cyclosporine levels	Drugs that raise cyclosporine levels
Isoniazid (INH)	Diltiazem
Rifampin	Verapamil
Ethambutol	Nicardipine
Dilantin	Erythromycin
Phenobarbital	Ketoconazole
Nafcillin	Metoclopramide
Ethanol	Cimetadine
Cholestyramine	Ranitidine
Octreotide	Ciprofloxacin
Sulfamethoxazole	

level suddenly changes, always look first for a new drug interaction before changing the cyclosporine dose. For example, during the winter season the frequent upper respiratory infections in these immunosuppressed patients are often treated with erythromycin by a local referring physician who does not realize the potent drug interaction that may double the cyclosporine level. Third, one cannot underestimate the importance of taking the cyclosporine dose with a meal containing some fat. A 50% increase in levels can be achieved by giving the same dose of drug after a fat meal or with a large glass of regular-fat milk. If patients are not careful about doing this regularly their levels will vary greatly and make management very difficult. Fourth, alterations in drug metabolism or absorption may occur as the result of specific clinical events so that dose changes must be modified by their course. For example, the patient gets CMV disease 10 weeks after transplantation and the resulting hepatitis decreases cyclosporine metabolism and the level increases significantly. Change the dose but remember to follow the level very carefully when the CMV infection resolves! The second example is viral gastroenteritis, which reduces the drug absorption. Our practice is to begin following levels carefully in any patient with more than 36 to 48 hours of diarrhea, nausea, or vomiting and we seriously consider an empiric dose increase. Should the use of intravenous cyclosporine be required (see above), the usual approach is to administer $\frac{1}{3}$ of the steady state oral dose by intravenous route over a 24-hour period.[78]

Cyclosporine Levels

Cyclosporine levels have received much discussion in the literature and at the present time there exist several different assays yielding very different numbers (Table 9.2).[80–84] Therefore, care must be taken not to confuse literature data from groups using different assays. Investigators argue about what is a therapeutic level, what is the best test, and if it is necessary to measure the intact drug alone or the metabolites. The critical point

TABLE 9.2. Cyclosporine drug levels.

Whole blood TDX[a] or RIA[b] (parent and metabolites)	500–800 ng/ml
Serum or plasma TDX or RIA (parent and metabolites)	250–400 ng/ml
Whole blood HPLC[c] (parent compound only)	250–350 ng/ml
Serum or plasma HPLC (parent compound only)	100–200 ng/ml
Serum monoclonal Ab[d] to CSA by RIA (parent compound only)	50–120 ng/ml

[a]TDX = fluorescent polarization technique.
[b]RIA = radioimmunoassay.
[c]HPLC = high-performance liquid chromatography.
[d]Ab = antibody.

is that each program should choose one test and validate the program's clinical experience over time. Unfortunately, there are no absolute therapeutic and toxic level ranges. The levels must be considered a guide and the therapy of each patient individualized with respect to the levels. In other words, a given patient will usually develop rejection or become toxic at the same level each time but these benchmarks will not be directly applicable to the next patient.

Complications

Table 9.3 lists the side effects of cyclosporine. Most of these effects are dose dependent and patients can be reassured that in time most problems will resolve or at least improve significantly. Immediately postoperatively the most common complication is hypertension (see Chapter 11). The addition of an angiotensin-converting enzyme inhibitor or a calcium antagonist (nifedipine) will significantly improve the hypertension control and permit almost every patient to be weaned off of nitroprusside. In the longer term most patients will tend to demonstrate higher morning blood pressures, which may reflect some tendency to salt retention on this drug that alters blood volume after a night in the supine position. Dietary salt restriction, a low-dose diuretic, and a conservative approach to changing antihypertensive drug doses based only on morning blood pressures is appropriate. Cyclosporine may cause seizures in the immediate postoper-

TABLE 9.3. Cyclosporine side effects.

Hypertension	Salt retention
Hyperglycemia	Hepatic toxicity
Extremity tremor	Hyperkalemia
Anxiety	Seizures
Insomnia	Conjunctivitis
Gingival hyperplasia	Acidosis (distal RTA[a])
Sensory paresthesias	Nephrotoxicity
Hirsutism	

[a]RTA = renal tubular acidosis.

ative period, typically in children and during intravenous administration. Over the longer term the patients may become tremulous, particularly with intentional fine motor movements like writing or eating. Many patients note mood and judgment alterations during the first 6 months when the doses and levels are high and we routinely warn the patients and the families to be careful and more understanding. A feeling of anxiety or malaise often occurs about 3 to 5 hours after the oral dose, which coincides with the peak absorption level. Finally, some patients demonstrate significant hyperkalemia and this must be followed closely. Cyclosporine impairs renal potassium excretion. Therefore, it is appropriate to urge dietary potassium control to all patients in the first 6 months after surgery. The addition of a diuretic, either a loop type (i.e., furosemide) or a thiazide, is effective in increasing renal potassium excretion and controlling this problem in most cyclosporine-treated patients.

Cyclosporine Nephrotoxicity

Cyclosporine nephrotoxicity is a universal problem in transplantation and begins in the first 24 hours after surgery and the initiation of this drug.[85] In fact, some programs have changed their protocols to avoid using cyclosporine until 5 to 7 days after surgery (see next section). In the authors' experience the key management strategy is to avoid diuretic use for the first 72 to 96 hours and prevent the patient from becoming intravascularly volume contracted [i.e., permit higher filling pressures, left arterial pressure (LAP) = 12–20 mmHg range]. Because postbypass patients typically third-space albumin and fluid extensively, they behave initially (12–72 hr) as if they are volume contracted. The addition of cyclosporine in the heart transplant patients results in renal vasoconstriction, which reduces the effective renal blood flow even further. Thus, urine output typically falls below 15 cc/hr during the first 24 to 36 hours postoperatively. This does not mean that the kidneys are not excreting most of the required urea nitrogen and creatinine, but rather that the urine is more concentrated. Unfortunately, many physicians intervene for more urine output by recommending loop diuretics despite the fact that the fall in urine volume is actually an appropriate response to the kidney's "interpretation" of the patient's volume status. When coupled with the potent cyclosporine-induced renal vasoconstriction the diuretic administration can result in renal shut-down or acute tubular necrosis (ATN) and complicate postoperative management significantly. In contrast, if the patient is left alone, after 72 to 96 hours the situation reverses, third space losses return to the circulation, and patients are often intravascular fluid overloaded and diuretic administration is appropriate and safe. Using this strategy in a series of more than 60 heart transplants, only a 6% postoperative incidence of renal failure was noted.

Cyclosporine nephrotoxicity is also a chronic problem. Almost all patients will demonstrate a reduced creatinine clearance and an elevated serum creatinine over the first weeks and months after the initiation of cyclosporine.[86] Nephrotoxicity and effective immunosuppression appear to be closely tied, just as in the case of azathioprine and bone marrow suppression. Therefore, it may not be appropriate to continue to decrease the cyclosporine dose based on an elevated creatinine level. Rather, by following the drug levels and serial endomyocardial biopsies, one should aim for a cyclosporine dose that spares the renal function as much as possible while maintaining a therapeutic drug level (Table 9.2) and preventing rejection. Fortunately, the nephrotoxicity usually stabilizes after 6 to 12 months, reflecting the lower cyclosporine levels required to prevent rejection at this point. In practice, many patients will have creatinine levels in the 1.8 to 2.5 mg% range during the first year. If the creatinine rises over 3.0 mg% the cyclosporine dose can usually be decreased safely. The possibility of nephrotoxicity from other drugs is also an important consideration since cyclosporine increases the risk significantly. Thus, drugs that rarely evidence toxicity in general practice may result in an elevated creatinine level in heart transplant patients. Common examples include the cephalosporins, nonsteroidal antiinflammatory agents, iodine radiocontrast agents, and trimethoprim/sulfamethoxazole. Finally, transplant patients are very sensitive to intravascular volume contraction. Excessive diuretic use or any febrile or gastrointestinal disorder that results in viremic symptoms (vasodilatation) and fluid loss will frequently be associated with a sharp rise in the serum creatinine.

Monoclonal and Polyclonal Antilymphocyte Antibodies

History

The first use of antilymphocyte serum to inhibit the immune response and alter the course of rejection was reported by Woodruff and Anderson in 1963.[87] This was followed with a clinical trial by Starzl and colleagues in 1967[88] and since then many reports have been published.[89–93] Antilymphocyte serum is made by immunizing animals, usually horses, rabbits, or goats, with human lymphocytes obtained from juvenile thymus glands (antithymocyte serum) or cadaver lymph nodes (antilymphocyte serum). The animals respond by generating many different antibodies against the foreign protein determinants or antigens expressed on the cell surfaces of these human cells. These antibodies are "harvested" by bleeding the animals and preparing the serum. Because these pooled serum preparations contain many different antibodies they are called "polyclonal". There are several limitations of these polyclonal preparations. First, the commercial availability of these preparations was inconsistent and expensive, so that many large centers (e.g., University of Minnesota) made their own and distributed these to other centers by special arrangement.

Second, the potency of the preparations varied from batch to batch and the efficacy varied from center to center. Third, it was difficult to use these preparations in large randomized trials because of these problems, thus limiting the analysis of their efficacy.

The Nobel prize-winning accomplishment of Kohler and Milstein was the development of the monoclonal antibody technique in 1975.[94] The immunization of mice with antigen is followed by the fusion of the mouse antibody-producing B cells with a malignant plasma cell line to create an immortal antibody-producing hybridoma. This hybridoma will only produce a single antibody of constant specificity and structure, called a "monoclonal" antibody. The ability to sort out the complex polyclonal antibody response to antigen into a set of monoclonal antibodies of unique specificities has profoundly changed immunology. One consequence of this development was the creation of a series of monoclonal anti-T cell antibodies, one of which is OKT3.[95] This antibody defines a protein on the T-cell surface that is associated with the T-cell antigen receptor, the CD3 molecule. The first clinical use of this antibody was reported by Cosimi and colleagues in 1981[96] to treat acute rejection in kidney transplant patients. Its efficacy in treating rejection in heart transplant patients was demonstrated next.[97] It is now also used commonly in induction or quadruple drug therapy, as will be described in the next section. Relative to the problems with the polyclonal antisera, the monoclonal antibody is always the same, can be produced in essentially limitless quantity forever, and each center will be using the same antibody.

Mechanisms

Antilymphocyte antibodies (polyclonal or monoclonal) work by binding T cells and eliminating them by two means: complement fixation with cell lysis and reticuloendothelial uptake in the liver and spleen by opsonization of the antibody-coated cells. In the case of murine monoclonal antibodies, the latter mechanism is thought to be dominant because there is no evidence for complement fixation and subsequent cell lysis. Therefore, the lymphocytes that are eliminated depend almost entirely on the target specificity of the antibodies given to the patient. In the case of the polyclonal antisera, there are many different antibodies present with a broad antilymphocyte reactivity. Lymphocytes may be bound by more than one antibody under these circumstances and this may enhance the efficacy of cell lysis and opsonization. In contrast, with a monoclonal antibody the lymphocyte is targeted for a single specificity. However, whether polyclonal or monoclonal, the administration of antibody results in a rapid (i.e., 24–48 hr) elimination of both circulating and graft-infiltrating lymphocytes.

In the case of OKT3, which is the only commercially available monoclonal antibody for transplantation, the target is the CD3 molecule. The CD3 molecule is a complex of several polypeptide chains that is expressed on the surface of only mature T cells and it is in physical contact with the T-cell antigen receptor. The binding of OKT3 to the T cell blocks the ability of the T-cell antigen receptor to bind its antigen, presumably by steric hinderance but also by stripping the CD3/T-cell receptor complex off the T-cell surface. Thus, the blocking of T-cell antigen recognition during OKT3 administration is a potent aspect of its activity. The binding of OKT3 antibody to the T lymphocyte also results in T-cell activation as if the T cell were exposed to its antigen. Though the activation of T cells by OKT3 has been used for experimental work, its significance in clinical situations is unclear. However, T-cell activation may result in cytokine release, specifically tumor necrosis factor (TNF), and this cytokine may cause some of the OKT3 side effects like fever, chills, and hypotension.

Clinical Use

Antilymphocyte globulins are administered intravenously and daily in all cases. The dose differs with the preparation but is expressed in mg protein/kg of patient. OKT3 is given as a 5-mg dose intravenously, without an adjustment for patient weight. Because of the potential for an allergic reaction to the antisera, most protocols call for a skin test to be administered before therapy. If there is no evidence of a wheal and flare reaction in 1 hour then the antibody can be given. Premedication of the patient with steroids, acetaminophen, and an antihistamine can reduce the incidence or at least the severity of the febrile reactions that typically follow antibody administration. In the case of OKT3 it is important to make sure the patient is not volume overloaded before therapy because this state has been associated with acute pulmonary edema after antibody administration, presumably caused by a cytokine-mediated capillary leak.[98]

Antibody administration for therapy or prophylaxis of acute rejection varies from 7 to 14 days depending on individual center protocols. During OKT3 therapy, the doses of concomitant immunosuppression (Cy A, azathioprine) are usually reduced in order to minimize the risk of infection.[99] However, the guidelines for drug dose reduction varies from center to center, and no definitive data are available. It is extremely important to make certain that cyclosporine levels are increased back to the therapeutic range before the OKT3 is stopped in order to prevent rebound rejection, a significant problem in the kidney transplant experience.[100] Therefore, the cyclosporine dose should be returned to maintenance levels (with frequent blood level monitoring) 3 to 4 days before discontinuing OKT3. If the target cyclosporine level is not achieved, an additional few days of OKT3 can be administered if necessary.

Complications

The acute onset of fever, chills, malaise, dyspnea, headache, and hypotension is typical after antilymphocyte antibody administration, although the intensity of these reactions varies greatly in individual patients and with different antibody preparations (in the case of the polyclonal antisera). Fortunately, this "first dose" reaction is much less the second day and usually not an issue after the third dose. In fact, many programs stop the premedication after the third dose. It is interesting that the experience with these first dose reactions is much less when the antibodies are used for rejection prophylaxis. The current reasoning is that when using OKT3 for rejection prophylaxis, this results in T-cell lysis early after transplantation and before any immune activation of these cells. In contrast, when the antibodies are given to patients with acute rejection the lysed cells have been activated and release a much greater load of inflammatory cytokines, such as TNF.

OKT3 has been associated with an aseptic meningitis syndrome, including a cerebrospinal fluid (CSF) pleocytosis.[101] This syndrome usually occurs after several doses and may persist until the OKT3 is stopped. Some patients will evidence a prolonged fever without other symptoms and it will continue until the OKT3 is stopped. It remains the physician's responsibility to exclude infectious causes for meningitis or fever in these patients. Finally, there is little argument that antilymphocyte antibodies increase the long-term incidence of CMV and herpes simplex virus (HSV) infections in transplant patients[102,103] though the increase is in the 5% to 15% range.

Re-Use of Antibodies

The use of an antilymphocyte antibody for induction or acute rejection therapy exposes the patient to a foreign protein and allows the possibility of developing an anti-antibody. The presence of such anti-antibodies may result in a severe serum sickness reaction if the original antibody preparation is re-administered. This is a common problem with the polyclonal antibodies and, in general, they are administered only once to each patient. An anti-antibody can also block the ability of the antilymphocyte antibody to bind the lymphocytes and, thus, eliminate the antibody's therapeutic value.[104] This problem has been well documented for OKT3.[105] The incidence of such anti-antibody formation after OKT3 is quite variable depending on the assay used; it ranges from as low as 20% to as high as 80%[106] However, the titers of anti-OKT3 antibodies are usually less than 1 : 100 and, thus, OKT3 can still be used safely.[107] Nonetheless, it is advised to monitor patients' circulating T cell numbers when starting a second course of OKT3. If the T cell numbers do not promptly fall to less than 10% of their original, then an increase of the OKT3 dose or a trial of steroid therapy may be indicated. It is possible to measure the anti-OKT3 antibody titers directly, but this test is not available in most centers and turn-around time for specimen test results usually is not acceptable. A few centers, usually those using OKT3 for rejection prophylaxis, measure the anti-OKT3 titers in all patients after about 4 weeks so that the information is available in case of a re-treatment need.

Immunosuppressive Protocols

Double Versus Triple Therapy

The use of cyclosporine and prednisone is commonly called double drug therapy and with the addition of azathioprine it is called triple drug therapy. The most common practice is triple drug therapy. This is rational from the immunomechanistic viewpoint because these drugs have overlapping and potentially synergistic mechanisms. However, data from multiple kidney transplant centers collected by the University of California, Los Angeles registry comparing double and triple drug therapy does not show any significant differences in 1-year graft survival.[108] Nonetheless, many renal transplant programs have adopted triple drug protocols exclusively. Furthermore, the move from double therapy to triple therapy in heart transplant immunosuppression appears to have a positive impact on survival.[63] In addition, the chance to manipulate three different drugs to obtain adequate immunosuppression and avoid individual differences in patient side effects makes a good argument for triple drug therapy in clinical practice.

Quadruple Drug Therapy

The addition of an antilymphocyte preparation to a triple drug therapy, either a polyclonal antisera or OKT3, is called quadruple drug therapy. The antilymphocyte antibody is given immediately after surgery and daily for 7 to 14 days depending on the individual center's protocol. Because this antibody therapy is initiated at the time of transplantation it is often called "induction" therapy. There are three potential advantages of induction therapy. First, the potent immunosuppression created by eliminating circulating T cells allows cyclosporine to be held until a week after surgery when many of the problems impacting on renal function have resolved. Many centers have noted a reduction in postoperative renal failure and hypertension with this protocol.[109,110] Second, the prompt onset of immunosuppression with these antibodies as compared to the several days it might take to achieve therapeutic cyclosporine and azathioprine levels might enhance the efficacy of immunosuppression and reduce the risk of rejection. In fact, there is little doubt that these antibodies reduce the incidence of acute rejection and increase the time to first rejection. Third, because this potent immunosuppression is created during the initial contact of the patient's immune system with the transplant, some investigators have implied that it might favor the development of suppressor cells or other tolerance-inducing mechanisms. In other words, induction therapy may have some long lasting effect on the immune response leading to increased graft survival. Unfortunately, there is no evidence to support this line of reasoning. As previously reported for renal transplantation[6] and based on data from The Registry of the International Society for Heart Transplantation (Fig. 9.2), long-term graft/patient

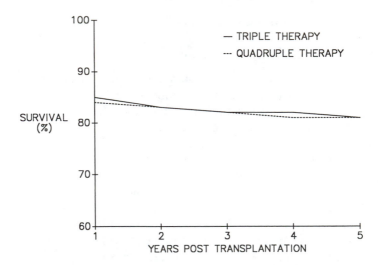

FIGURE 9.2. Data analyzed from The Registry of the International Society for Heart Transplantation that demonstrates no difference in patient survival between those patients receiving triple therapy immunosuppression (cyclosporine, azathioprine, prednisone) and those receiving quadruple therapy immunosuppression (triple therapy plus antilymphocyte antibodies). These data represent a total of 6578 patients in the triple therapy group and 3921 patients in the quadruple therapy group. The data for this graph was kindly provided by Dr. Michael P. Kaye.

survival is not changed by the use of induction therapy with antilymphocyte antibodies.[111]

There are several problems with quadruple drug therapy. A major issue is expense. Regardless of the agent used, the use of an antilymphocyte antibody preparation adds $4,000 to 7,000 to the cost of the transplant, excluding any increase in total hospital days that might also be added. Many programs have reported a modest increase in the incidence of viral infections after the use of antilymphocyte therapy, although this can be reduced if the other drugs are kept at lower doses and the period of induction therapy is decreased toward 7 days. Nonetheless, if there is no change in long term graft survival we must question the routine use of these agents. Is a reduction in the early incidence of rejection enough to balance the cost and infection problems? This remains a point of controversy and individual centers must consider their experience and decide.

Steroid-Free Protocols

In the last several years a number of programs have reported their success in avoiding the long-term use of steroids.[112,113] The advantages are obvious and these programs have confirmed a reduction in lipoprotein abnormalities, hypertension, and other classic steroid side effects. Although a number of protocols have been reported, the common ground is the use of induction therapy with an antilymphocyte antibody preparation. Most programs will use low-dose steroids for a short time after surgery and then rapidly wean and discontinue the drug. The incidence of recurrent rejection requiring the re-institution of steroids differs in each center but approximately 30% of patients will fail the attempt.[114] Nonetheless, most of these patients are just started back on prednisone after the rejection is treated successfully and, thus, it can be argued that the risk to the patient is low. Unfortunately, it is too soon to determine the long-term survival of patients and particularly the incidence of accelerated atherosclerosis in the steroid-free patients.

Treatment of Acute Rejection

Rejection represents a failure of immunosuppression to prevent the immune response from mobilizing the effector cells required to mediate tissue injury. This is a key concept to remember for two clinical reasons. First, the clinician should always ask *why* did the patient reject at any given point. Sometimes the patient's cyclosporine level has fallen below the therapeutic level, for example, because of a drug interaction, an over-adjustment in dose, or noncompliance. These issues must be identified and addressed or rejection therapy will be ineffective. Sometimes rejection is associated with an episode of CMV infection. This is usually a complex situation in which the patient has been very ill, azathioprine has usually been stopped because of severe leukopenia, and then as the patient recovers he suddenly evidences rejection on the biopsy. These patients should be treated cautiously because there is a real risk of reactivating the CMV illness. Second, the clinician must always remember that the patient is on immunosuppressive drug therapy when rejection is diagnosed. Therefore, antirejection therapy is superimposed on the immunosuppression baseline. One can take advantage of this fact because sometimes a simple adjustment of the cyclosporine or azathioprine doses may successfully treat a mild rejection. Furthermore, many centers may not treat a patient with mild rejection at all, especially if the patient is remote from transplantation and clinically stable. In contrast, there is a population of patients who, despite repeated courses of rejection therapy, continue to have evidence of mild or early moderate rejection. It is conceivable that these patients will eventually succumb to chronic rejection but that repeated antirejection therapies will only make them ill. One can hope that in the future, with the institution of alternative immunosuppressive strategies or new drugs, that these "chronic triple drug failures" may be treated effectively.

Corticosteroids

Corticosteroids for rejection can be used intravenously as methylprednisolone in much the same way they are used immediately posttransplant.

The usual therapy is 1 gm methylprednisolone each day for 3 consecutive days. Based on the authors' experience, it appears that one can tailor the amount of corticosteroids given to the intensity of the rejection episode as well as the patient's time from transplantation. For instance, successful rejection therapy can be achieved with only 500 mg/day in patients with more mild rejection or patients with rejection presenting more than 3 months posttransplant, and we have used as little as 250 mg/day for 5 days in patients with rejection in the face of a resolving CMV infection or some other infectious complication.

Corticosteroids can also be given orally to treat rejection.[115] In fact, there is no evidence that intravenous steroids are more effective than oral. In patients without hemodynamic compromise, a short oral pulse of prednisone, 100 mg for 5 days can be tried before turning to more aggressive therapy.

The complications of pulse steroid therapy are essentially the same as postoperative problems, including hyperglycemia, hypertension, fluid retention, altered judgment, anxiety, and sleep disturbances. The infection risk is higher after pulse steroids in patients within 2 to 4 months of surgery because this coincides with the peak incidence of CMV and other opportunistic infections. In other words, a patient who might otherwise have manifested a clinically asymptomatic CMV antibody titer rise might present with active CMV disease after a steroid pulse. Finally, patients have complained of blurred vision after pulse steroids, which resolves spontaneously within two weeks. If blurred vision persists, we suggest an expert retinal exam to exclude CMV retinitis. Another cause of blurred vision after a steroid pulse is severe hyperglycemia.

Antilymphocyte Antibodies

Antilymphocyte antibodies have been previously discussed for induction or quadruple drug therapy and they can also be used to treat acute rejection. The primary decision is *when* to use these drugs in relation to the use of corticosteroids. The most conservative position is to reserve these agents for steroid failures. This is supported by several arguments. First, the antilymphocyte antibodies are very expensive. A typical course of antibodies will cost approximately $5,000, not including hospitalization or out-patient facility fees, whereas a course of intravenous steroids costs less than $200. Second, the use of antilymphocyte antibodies will increase the risk of infectious complications, particularly CMV infection. Third, the use of these agents is not flexible. There is no way to give intermediate doses such as previously suggested for the steroids. One approach is to use a modified or low-dose steroid pulse first, a full-dose steroid course next, and reserve antilymphocyte antibody therapy for these failures. With this approach antilymphocyte antibody therapy has been used sparingly at the authors' institution (only two courses in 65 consecutive patients) with excellent graft survival and a very low incidence of CMV and other opportunistic infections.

Another approach is to use antilymphocyte therapy liberally. This is based on several arguments. First, these agents are powerful and therapy success is better than 90% with a single course. Second, prompt reversal of rejection may spare cardiac injury that could alter cardiac function or reserve in the long term. Third, the use of these agents might enhance the development of long term transplant success by first profoundly depleting T cells and then permitting them to redevelop after the transplant has been in place. This argument is based on evidence in irradiated and thymectomized animal models which suggests that when T-cell numbers recover from the drug-induced depletion, they accept the graft as "self," and, thus, do not cause rejection. Unfortunately, there is no evidence to support this theory in current clinical practice with antilymphocyte therapy.

The choice of using a polyclonal antilymphocyte sera or using the monoclonal OKT3 is largely based on the center's preference and on availability of reagents. Both types of preparation appear to be equally effective on clinical grounds. However, the commercial availability of OKT3 and the large body of data on its use for rejection have made this reagent the choice of most programs. The use of OKT3 for rejection is essentially the same as that for induction therapy. A course of OKT3 is usually for 10 to 14 days, though some centers have been experimenting with a 7-day course. Most centers will measure circulating T-cell numbers (by flow cytometry) at least once during the initiation of therapy to confirm that the therapy is successful. The centers that use OKT3 for induction therapy have an additional concern, which is the development of anti-OKT3 antibodies. This has been discussed earlier.

Other Agents

If one considers the basic concept that rejection represents the failure of the baseline immunosuppression, one understands the basis by which some centers add methotrexate[115] or substitute cytoxan for azathioprine when rejection is recurrent despite adequate therapy. However, the experience with these regimens remains limited to a few centers, the trials have been neither prospective nor randomized, and historically such maneuvers have not been successful in renal transplantation. Nonetheless, the initial reports are promising.

Future Directions

New Monoclonal Antibodies

The current monoclonal antibody, OKT3, is directed against the CD3 complex of the T-cell antigen receptor, which is expressed by virtually all circulating or mature T cells. Therefore, one limitation of this agent is the nonselective removal of all T cells and, thus, significant risk of infection. The objective of new antibody reagents is a more selective targeting of only the T cells involved in recognition of the graft. One such reagent that has been used in several preliminary clinical trials with some encouraging success is directed at the IL-2 receptor.[116] The expression of IL-2 receptors by T cells is an early event that follows immune activation and it is restricted to those T-cell clones that recognize the transplanted organ as foreign. Thus, removal of these early activated T cells would be both powerful and relatively selective. There are three practical problems. First, the IL-2 receptor is a complex of two protein chains and this antibody is binding to only one, the 55-kDa light chain. The heavier 75-kDa chain of the receptor can bind IL-2, though with a lower affinity than the intact complex of two chains, and activate the T cell without the presence of the 55-kDa chain. Therefore, if the cell is stripped of the 55-kDa chains by the antibody the T cells can still bind and respond to IL-2. Second, the removal of T cells by monoclonal antibodies depends on cell coating followed either by reticuloendothelial cell uptake or complement-mediated lysis. Unfortunately, both these mechanisms depend on the quantity of antibody on the cell surface, which decreases significantly after the first few days of therapy because the target surface molecules have been stripped away. Third, the blockade of the immune response by the anti-IL-2 receptor antibody is only present while the antibody is being infused and the T cells can re-express their IL-2 receptors within several hours of the antibody's disappearance. Although it was hoped that early removal of the responding T cell clones would result in permanent acceptance of the transplant, this has not occurred in the experimental systems studied.

The development of a monoclonal antibody against the 75-kDa chain might address the first problem and avoid T-cell activation by the 75-kDa chain acting alone. However, the second problem represents a major problem for any monoclonal antibody strategy. They can only be administered intravenously and for relatively short periods of time before they are neutralized by anti-antibodies produced by the patient. When antibody therapy is discontinued the T cells can quickly re-express these surface molecules and the immune system has another opportunity to recognize the transplant as foreign and cause rejection. Monoclonal antibodies against helper T cells or killer T cells are also available and effective in certain experimental models although they have not yet been used in patients. Still, they will only be useful to treat acute rejection as pulse or induction therapy until we figure out a strategy to alter the basic dynamics of the long-term immune response.

Hybrid Molecules

One strategy to alter the immune response for the long term is to eliminate the population of activated T-cell clones more effectively than by coating them with antibody and relying on the reticuloendothelial and complement systems to remove the cells. T cells that bind a cytokine (such as IL-2) to their receptors will also internalize the IL-2 molecule. Thus, investigators have used molecular engineering technology to couple the IL-2 molecule with a potent cellular toxin from diphtheria.[117] When the T cells bind this hybrid IL-2/toxin they are killed directly, and experimental evidence in the rat model has shown that heart transplant success can be enhanced.[118] Another version of this strategy has been coupling monoclonal antibodies with the plant toxin ricin. Again, the binding of antibody results in internalization of the antibody carrying its toxin conjugate and the T cell is directly eliminated. Unfortunately, this area is still experimental and it remains to be seen whether this will result in long-term alteration of the immune response.

Total Lymphoid Irradiation

Total lymphoid irradiation (TLI) has been used in experimental models for a long time and results in permanent alterations in circulating T cell populations. In most experimental transplant models the use of TLI results in permanent graft tolerance without the use of immunosuppressive drugs. It has also been used by investigators in human kidney transplantation, where it has reduced the incidence of rejection in the first year. However, it is too early to assess its part in improving long-term function.[119] In these human patients a reduction in the number of circulating helper T cells was found as long as 1 year after TLI, which suggests that this strategy does indeed affect the immune response in the long term. It is also unclear whether TLI will increase the risk of malignancy, particularly lymphoma or leukemia.

New Drugs: FK506 and Rapamycin

Two new fungal derivatives, FK506 and rapamycin, both of which are lipophilic macrolides made from the streptomyces family of fungi,[120,121] have been potent in animal models of transplantation. FK506 has now been used in humans in liver, kidney, and pancreas transplantation with encouraging initial results.[122]

Whether these drugs can replace cyclosporine or can be added as additional therapy is currently unclear. Furthermore, it is important to note that the success of these new drugs in the animal models is no more impressive than that of cyclosporine. Therefore, there is no a priori reason to expect that these drugs will be better than cyclosporine in human patients. The fact that these agents have different side effect profiles may be most important because it has already been noted that the problems associated with cyclosporine, nephrotoxicity and hypertension, limit the full use of this drug in practice. However, whereas neither FK506 or rapamycin show evidence of nephrotoxicity, FK506 was poorly tolerated by animals in many of the early experiments, due to anorexia, neurotoxicity, liver toxicity, and an acute vasculitis in dogs. On the other hand, the early reports suggest that the human patients have tolerated FK506 better than the animals.

There are several other new drugs being studied in the animal models. These include deoxyspergualin, RS 61443, thalidomide, prostaglandin metabolites, purine metabolism inhibitors, and others. Therefore, the future holds considerable promise for the development of newer, more effective, and less toxic immunosuppressive protocols.

References

1. Bieber CP, Hunt SA, Schwinn DA, et al. Complications in long-term survivors of cardiac transplantation. *Transplant Proc*. 1981;13:207–211.
2. Uretsky BF, Murali S, Reddy PS, et al. Development of coronary artery disease in cardiac tranplant patients receiving immunosuppressive therapy with cyclosporine and prednisone. *Circulation*. 1987;76:827–834.
3. Billingham ME. Cardiac transplant atherosclerosis. *Tranplant Proc*. 1987;19(suppl 5):19–25.
4. Gao SZ, Alderman EL, Schroeder JS, et al. Accelerated coronary vascular disease in the heart transplant patient: coronary arteriographic findings. *J Am Coll Cardiol*. 1988;12:334–340.
5. Johnson DE, Gao SZ, Schroeder JS, et al. The spectrum of coronary artery pathologic findings in human cardiac allografts. *J Heart Transplant*. 1989;8:349–359.
6. The North Italy Transplant Program (NITP). Factors influencing cadaver kidney tranplantation outcome in the cyclosporine era. In: Teraski P, ed. *Clinical Transplants 1988*. Los Angeles, Calif: UCLA Tissue Typing Laboratory; 1988:131–145.
7. Schwartz R, Dameshek W. Drug induced immunological tolerance. *Nature*. 1959; 1983:1682–1683.
8. Calne RY. Rejection of renal homografts: inhibition in dogs by 6-mercatopurine. *Lancet*. 1960;1:417–418.
9. Calne RY, Alexandre GP, Murray JE. A study of the effects of drugs in prolonging survival of homologous renal transplants in dogs. *Ann NY Acad Sci*. 1962;99:743–761.
10. Elion GB. Pharmacologic and physical agents. Immunosuppressive agents. *Transplant Proc*. 1975;9:975–979.
11. Murray JE, Merrill JP, Harrison JH, et al. Prolonged survival of human kidney homografts by immunosuppressive therapy. *N Engl J Med*. 1963;268:1315–1323.
12. Woodruff MFA, Robson JS, Nolan B, et al. Homotransplantation of kidney in patients treated by preoperative local irradiation and postoperative administration of an antimetabolite (Imuran): report of six cases. *Lancet*. 1963;2:675–682.
13. Starzl TE, Marchioro TL, Waddel WR. The reversal of rejection in human

renal homografts with subsequent development of homograft tolerance. *Surg Gynecol Obstet*. 1963;117:385–395.

14. Hume DM, Magee JH, Kauffman HM, et al. Renal homotransplantation in man in modified recipients. *Ann Surg*. 1963;158:608–644.

15. McCormack JJ, Johns DG. Purine antimetabolites. In: Chabner B, ed. *Pharmacologic Principles of Cancer Treatment*. Philadelphia, Penn: WB Saunders Co; 1982:213–228.

16. Jensen MK. Chromosome studies in patients treated with azathioprine and amethopterin. *Acta Med Scand*. 1967;182:445–455.

17. Old CW, Flannery EP, Grogan TM, et al. Azathioprine-induced pure red cell aplasia. *JAMA*. 1978;240:552–554.

18. Bennett WM, Norman DJ. Maintenance immunosuppression: azathioprine and glucocorticoids. In: Milford, EL, ed. *Renal Transplantation*. New York, NY: Churchill Livingstone; 1989:97–103.

19. Sieber SM, Adamson RH. Toxicity of antineoplastic agents in man: chromosomal aberrations, antifertility effects, congenital malformations and carcinogenic potential. *Adv Cancer Res*. 1975;22:57–155.

20. Gilmore IT, Holden G, Rodan KS. Acute leukemia during azathioprine therapy. *Postgrad Med J*. 1977;53:173–174.

21. Scharf J, Nahir M, Eidelman S, et al. Carcinoma of the bladder with azathioprine therapy. *JAMA*. 1977;237:152.

22. Kaplan SR, Calabresi P. Immunosuppressive agents. *N Engl J Med*. 1973;289:1234–1236.

23. Herskowitz LJ, Olansky S, Lang PG. Acute pancreatitis associated with long-term azathioprine therapy. *Arch Dermatol*. 1979;115:179.

24. Foster GL, Smith PE. Hypophysectomy and replacement therapy in relation to basal metabolism and specific dynamic action in the rat. *JAMA*. 1926;87:2151–2153.

25. Li CH, Evans HM, Simpson ME. Adrenocorticotrophic hormone. *J Biol Chem*. 1943;149:413–424.

26. Sayers G, White A, Long CNH. Preparation and properties of pituitary adrenocorticotrophic hormone. *J Biol Chem*. 1943;149:425–436.

27. Bell PH, Howard KS, Shephard RG, et al. Studies with corticotrophin II. Pepsin degradation of Beta-corticotrophin. *J Am Chem Soc*. 1956;78:5059–5066.

28. Schwyzer R, Seibert P. Total synthesis of adrenocorticotrophic hormone. *Nature*. 1963;199:172–174.

29. tbMerrill JP, Murray JE, Harrison JH, et al. Successful homotransplantation of the kidney between nonidentical twins. *N Engl J Med*. 1960;262:1251–1260.

30. Goodwin WE, Mims MM, Kaufman JJ. Human renal transplantation III: technical problems encoutered in six cases of kidney homotransplantation. *Trans Am Assoc Genitourin Surg*. 1962;54:116–125.

31. Durum SK, Schmidt JA, Oppenheim JJ. Interleukin-1: an immunological perspective. *Annu Rev Immunol*. 1985;3:263–288.

32. MacDonald HR, Habholz MT. T-cell activation. *Annu Rev Cell Biol*. 1986;2:231–253.

33. Smith KA. Interleukin-2: inception, impact, and implications. *Science*. 1988;240:1169–1176.

34. Van Snick J, Vink A, Cayphas S, et al. Interleukin-HPl, a T cell-derived

hybridoma growth factor that supports the in vitro growth of murine plasma-cytomas. *J Exper Med*. 1987;165:641–649.

35. Cantrell DA, Smith KA. The interleukin-2 T-cell system: a new cell growth model. *Science*. 1984;224:1312–1316.

36. Sandvig S, Laskay T, Anderson J, et al. Gamma-interferon produced by CD3+ and CD3− lymphocytes. *Immunol Rev*. 1987;97:51–65.

37. Tsai WY, Carlstedt-Duke J, Weigel NL, et al. Molecular interactions of steroid hormone receptor with its enhancer element: evidence for receptor dimer formation. *Cell*. 1988;55:361–369.

38. Yamamoto KR. Steroid receptor regulated transcription of specific genes and gene networks. *Annu Rev Genet*. 1985;19:209–252.

39. Russell SW, Salomon DR. Macrophage effector and regulatory functions. In: Reif AE, Mitchell MS, eds. *Immunity to Cancer*. New York, NY: Academic Press, 1985:205–216.

40. Hall BM, Dorsch SW. Cells mediating allograft rejection. *Immunol Rev*. 1984;77:31–79.

41. Soyka LF, Saxena KM. Alternate day steroid therapy for nephrotic children. *JAMA*. 1965;192:225–230.

42. Harter JC, Reddy WJ, Thorn GW. Studies on an intermittent corticosteroid dosage regimen. *N Engl J Med*. 1963;269:591–596.

43. Dumler F, Levin NW, Szego G, et al. Long-term alternate day steroid therapy in renal transplantation. *Transplantation*. 1982;34:78–82.

44. Lippman ME, Eil C. Steroid therapy of cancer. In: Chabner B, ed. *Pharmacologic Principles of Cancer Treatment*. Philadelphia, Penn: WB Saunders Co; 1982:141–143.

45. d'Apice AJF. Non-specific immunosuppression: azathioprine and steroids. In: Morris PJ, ed. *Kidney Transplantation: Principles and Practice*. Orlando, Fla: Grune & Stratton Inc; 1984:251–256.

46. Renlund DG, Bristow MR, Crandall BG, et al. Hypercholesterolemia after heart transplantation: amelioration by corticosteroid-free maintenance immunosuppression. *J Heart Transplant*. 1989;8:214–220.

47. Merion RM, White DJG, Thiru S, et al. Cyclosporine: five years' experience in cadaveric renal transplantaiton. *N Engl J Med*. 1984;310:148–154.

48. El-Shaboury AH, Hayes TM. Hyperlipidaemia in asthmatic patients on long-term steroid therapy. *Br Med J*. 1973;2:85–86.

49. Ibels LS, Alfrey AC, Weil R. Hyperlipidemia in adult,   pediatric and diabetic renal transplant recipients. *Am J Med*. 1978;64:634–642.

50. Ettinger WH, Applebaum-Bowden D, Goldbert AP, et al. Dyslipoproteinemia in systemic lupus erythematosus. *Am J Med*. 1987;83:503–508.

51. Borel JF, Feurer C, Bugler HU, et al. Biological effects of cyclosporin A: a new antilymphocytic agent. *Agents Actions*. 1976;6:468–475.

52. Borel JF, Feurer C, Magnee C, et al. Effects of the new anti-lymphocytic peptide cyclosporin A in animals. *Immunology*. 1977;32:1017–1025.

53. Borel JF. The history of cyclosporin A and its significance. In: White DJG, ed. *Cyclosporin A: Proceedings of an International Conference on Cyclosporin A*. Amsterdam: Elsevier Biomedical Press; 1982:5–17.

54. Kostakis AJ, White DJG, Calne RY. Prolongation of rat heart allograft survival by cyclosporin A. *IRCS J Med Sci*. 1977;5:280–284.

55. Calne RY, White DJG. Cyclosporin A: a powerful immunosuppressant in dogs with renal allografts. *IRCS J Med Sci*. 1977;5:595–601.
56. Green CJ, Allison AC, Rolles K. Prolonged survival of pig orthotopic heart grafts treated with cyclosporin A. *Lancet*. 1978;1:1182–1183.
57. Calne RY, Rolles K, White DJG, et al. Cyclosporin A initially as the only immunosuppressant in 34 recipients of cadaveric organs: 32 kidneys, 2 pancreases and 2 livers. *Lancet*. 1979;2:1033–1036.
58. Calne RY, Rolles K, White DJG, et al. Cyclosporin-A in clinical organ grafting. *Transplant Proc*. 1981;13:349–358.
59. Calne RY, White DJG. The use of cyclosporin A in clinical organ grafting. *Ann Surg*. 1982;196:330–337.
60. Canadian Multicentre Transplant Study Group. A randomized clinical trial of cyclosporine in cadaveric renal transplantation: analysis at three years. *N Engl J Med*. 1986;314:1219–1225.
61. Johnson RWG. Cyclosporine in cadaveric renal transplantation: three year follow-up of European multicentre trial. *Transplant Proc*. 1986;18:1229–1233.
62. White DJG. Immunosuppression for cardiac transplantation. In: Wallwork J, ed. *Heart and Heart-Lung Transplantation*. Philadelphia, Penn: WB Saunders Co; 1989:163.
63. Shumway SJ, Kaye MP. The international society for heart transplantation registry. In: Terasaki P, ed. *Clinical Transplant 1988*. Los Angeles, Calif: UCLA Tissue Typing Laboratory; 1988:1–5.
64. Hess AD, Tutschka PJ, Santos GW. The effect of cyclosporin A on T-lymphocyte subpopulations. In: White DJG, ed. *Cyclosporin A: Proceedings of an International Conference on Cyclosporin A*. Amsterdam: Elsevier Biomedical Press; 1982:209–231.
65. Cohen DJ, Loertscher R, Rubin MF, et al. Cyclosporine: a new immunosuppressive agent for organ transplantation. *Ann Intern Med*. 1984;101:667–682.
66. Kalman VK, Klimpel GR. Cyclosporin A inhibits the production of gamma interferon (IFN gamma) but does not inhibit production of virus induced IFN alpha/beta. *Cell Immunol*. 1983;78:122–129.
67. Reem GH, Cook LA, Vilcek J. Gamma interferon synthesis by human thymocytes and T lymphocytes inhibited by cyclosporin A. *Science*. 1983;222:63–65.
68. Culpepper J, Lee F. Glucocorticoid regulation of lymphokine production by murine T-lymphocytes. In: Webb DR, Goeddel DV, eds. *Lymphokines*. Orlando, Fla: Academic Press; 1987;13:275–289.
69. Grey HM, Chestnut R. Antigen processing and presentation to T cells. *Immunol Today*. 1985;6:101–106.
70. Mayer T, Fuller A, Fuller T, et al. Characterization of in vivo activated allospecific T lymphocytes propagated from human renal allograft biopsies undergoing rejection. *J Immunol*. 1985;134:258–264.
71. Balkwill FK, Burke F. The cytokine network. *Immunol Today*. 1989;10:299–304.
72. Kronke M, Leonard WJ, Depper JM, et al. Cyclosporin A inhibits T-cell growth factor gene expression at the level of mRNA transcription. *Proc Natl Acad Sci USA*. 1984;81:5214–5218.

73. Handschumacher RE, Harding M, Rice J, et al. Cyclophilin: a specific cytosolic binding protein for cyclosporin A. *Science*. 1984;226:544–546.
74. Emmel EA, Verweij CL, Durand DB, et al. Cyclosporine specifically inhibits function of nuclear proteins involved in T cell activities. *Science*. 1989;246:1617–1620.
75. Fischer G, Wittmann-Leibold B, Lang K, et al. Cyclophilin and peptidyl-proyl cis-trans isomerase are probably identical proteins. *Nature*. 1989;337:476–478.
76. Kahan BD, Ried M, Newberger J. Pharmacokinetics of cyclosporine in human renal transplantation. *Transplant Proc*. 1983;15:446–453.
77. Keown PA, Stiller CR, Sinclair NR, et al. The clinical relevance of cyclosporine blood levels as measured by radioimmunoassay. *Transplant Proc* 1983;15(no.4, suppl 1):2438–2441.
78. Kahan BD. Immunosuppressive therapy with cyclosporine for cardiac transplantation. *Circulation*. 1987;75:40–50.
79. Kahan BD. Cyclosporine: a powerful addition to the immunosuppressive armamentarium. *Am J Kidney Dis*. 1984;3:444–455.
80. Faynor SM, Moyer TP, Sterioff S. Therapeutic drug monitoring of cyclosporine. *Mayo Clin Proc*. 1984;59:571–572.
81. Burkle WS. Cyclosporine pharmacokinetics and blood level monitoring. *Drug Intell Clin Pharm*. 1985;19:101–105.
82. Robinson WT, Schran HF, Barry EP. Methods to measure cyclosporine levels—high pressure liquid chromatography, radioimmunoassay, and correlation. *Transplant Proc*. 1983;156(no. 4, suppl 1):2403–2408.
83. Donatsch P, Abisch E, Homberger M, et al. A radioimmunoassay to measure cyclosporin A in plasma and serum samples. *J Immunoassay*. 1981;2:19–32.
84. NACB/AACC Task Force on Cyclosporine Monitoring. Critical issues in cyclosporine monitoring. *Clin Chem*. 1987;33:1269.1288.
85. McGiffin DC, Kirklin JK, Naftel DC. Acute renal failure after heart transplantation and cyclosporine therapy. *J Heart Transplant*. 1985;4:396–399.
86. Moran M, Tomlanovich S, Myers BD. Cyclosporine-induced chronic nephropathy in human recipients of cardiac allografts. *Transplant Proc*. 1985;17(no. 4, suppl 1):185–190.
87. Woodruff MF, Anderson NA. Effect of lymphocyte depletion by thoracic duct fistula and antilymphocytic serum on the survival of skin homografts in rats. *Nature*. 1963;200:702–704.
88. Starzl TE, Porter KA, Iwasaki Y. Antilymphocytic serum in renal transplantation. In: Wolstenhome GRW, O'Connor M, eds. *Antilymphoctic Serum*. CIBA study Group No. 29. Boston, Mass: Little Brown & Co; 1967:4.
89. Sheil AGR, Kelly GE, Storey BG, et al. Controlled clinical trial of antilymphocyte globulin in patients with renal allografts from cadaver donors. *Lancet*. 1971;1:359–363.
90. Taylor HE, Ackman CFD, Horowitz I. Canadian clinical trial of antilymphocyte globulin in human cadaver renal transplantation. *Can Med Assoc J*. 1976;115:1205–1208.
91. Launois B, Campion JP, Faucher R, et al. Prospective randomized clinical trial in patients with cadaver-kidney transplants. *Transplant Proc*. 1977;9:1027–1030.
92. Butt KMH, Zielinski CM, Parsa I. Trends in immunosuppression for kidney transplantation. *Kidney Int*. 1978;13:S95–98.

93. Wechter WJ, Brodie JA, Morrell RM. Antithymocyte globulin (ATGAM) in renal allograft recipients. Multicenter trials using a 14-dose regimen. *Transplantation*. 1979;28:294–302.
94. Kohler G, Milstein C. Continuous cultures of fused cells secreting antibody of predefined specificity. *Nature*. 1975;256:495–497.
95. Kung PC, Goldstein G, Reinherz EL, et al. Monoclonal antibodies defining distinctive human T cell surface antigens. *Science*. 1979;206:347–349.
96. Cosimi AB, Burton RC, Colvin RB. Treatment of acute renal allograft rejection wiht OKT3 antibody. *Transplantation*. 1981;32:535–539.
97. Bristow MR, Gilbert EM, Renlund DG, et al. Use of OKT3 in heart transplantation; review of the initial experience. *Transplant Proc*. 1988;7:1–11.
98. Goldstein G, Schindler J, Sheahan M, et al. Orthoclone OKT3 treatment of acute renal allograft rejection. *Transplant Proc*. 1985;17:129–131.
99. Rubin RH, Cosimi AB, Hirsch MS, et al. Effects of antithymocyte globulin on cytomegalovirus infection in renal transplant recipients. *Transplantation*. 1981;31:143–145.
100. Delmonico FL, Auchincloss H, Rubin RH, et al. The selective use of anti-lymphocyte serum for cyclosporine treated patients with renal allograft dysfunction. *Ann Surg*. 1987;206:649–654.
101. Martin MA, Massanari M, Nghiem DD, et al. Nosocomial aseptic menigitis associated with administration of OKT3. *JAMA*. 1988;259:2002–2005.
102. Pass RF, Whitley RJ, Diethelm AG, et al. Cytomegalovirus infection in patients with renal transplants. Potentiation by antithymocyte globulin and an incompatible graft. *J Infect Dis*. 1980;142:9–17.
103. Pass RF, Whitley RJ, Welchel JD, et al. Identification of patients with increased risk of infection with herpes simplex virus after renal transplantation. *J Infect Dis*. 1979;140:487–492.
104. Delmonico F, Tolkhoff-Rubin N. Treatment of acute rejection. In: Milford E, ed. *Renal Transplantation*. New York, NY: Churchill Livingstone; 1989:129–146.
105. Goldstein G, Fuccelli AJ, Norman DJ, et al. OKT3 monoclonal antibody plasma levels during therapy and the subsequent development of host antibodies to OKT3. *Transplantation*. 1986;42:507–514.
106. Shield CF, Fucello AJ, Marlett R, et al. Human antibody response to anti-lymphocytic preparations in renal transplant patients. *Transplant Proc*. 1987;19:2217–2218.
107. Mayes JT, Thistlethwaite JR, Stuart JK, et al. Re-exposure to OKT3 in renal allograft recipients. *Transplantation*. 1988;45:349–353.
108. The North Italy Transplant Program (NITP). Factors influencing cadaver kidney transplantation outcome in the cyclosporine era. In: Terasaki P, ed. *Clinical Transplants 1988*. Los Angeles, Calif: UCLA Tissue Typing Laboratory; 1988:131–145.
109. Macris MP, Van Buren CT, Sweeney MS, et al. Selective use of OKT3 in heart transplantation with the use of risk factor analysis. *J Heart Transplant*. 1989;8:296–302.
110. Bristow MR, Gilbert EM, Renlund DG, et al. Use of OKT3 monoclonal antibody in heart transplantation: review of the initial experience. *J Heart Transplant*. 1988;7:1–11.

111. Kaye MP. International Heart Transplant Registry. Personal communication.
112. Katz MR, Barnhart GR, Szentpetery S, et al. Are steroids essential for successful maintenance of immunosuppression in heart transplantation? *J Heart Transplant*. 1987;6:293–297.
113. Esmore DS, Spratt PM, Keogh AM, et al. Cyclosporine and azathioprine immunosuppression without maintenance steroids: a prospective randomized trial. *J Heart Transplant*. 1989;8:194–199.
114. Renlund DG, O'Connell JB, Gilbert EM, et al. Feasibility of discontinuation of corticosteroid maintenance therapy in heart transplantation. *J Heart Transplant*. 1987;6:71–78.
115. Costanzo-Nordin MR, Grusk BB, Silver MA, et al. Reversal of recalcitrant cardiac allograft rejection with methotrexate. *Circulation*. 1988;78(suppl III): III-47–III-57.
116. Kupiec-Weglinski JW, Diamantstein T, Tilney NL. Interleukin 2 receptor-targeted therapy: rationale and applications in organ transplantation. *Transplantation*. 1988;46:785–792.
117. William DP, Parker K, Bacha P. Diphtheria toxin receptor binding domain substitution with interleukin 2: genetic construction and properties of a diphtheria toxin-related interleukin 2 fusion protein. *Protein Engineer*. 1987;1:493–500.
118. Kirkman RL, Bacha P, Barrett LV, et al. Prolongation of cardiac allograft survival in murine recipients treated with a diphtheria toxin-related interleukin-2 fusion protein. *Transplantation*. 1989;47:327–330.
119. Strober S, Dhillon M, Schubert M, et al. Acquired immune tolerance to cadaveric renal allografts: a study of three patients treated with total lymphoid irradiation. *N Engl J Med*. 1989;321:28–33.
120. Sawada S, Suzuki G, Kawase Y, et al. Novel immunosuppressive agent, FK506: in vitro effects on the cloned T-cell activation. *J Immunol*. 1987;139:1797–1803.
121. Calne RY, Collier DStJ, Lim S, et al. Rapamycin for immunosuppression in organ allografting. *Lancet*. 1989;2:227–228.
122. Starzl TE, Todo S, Fung J, et al. FK506 for liver, kidney and pancreas transplantation. *Lancet*. 1989;2:1000–1004.

10
Physiology and Hemodynamic Assessment of the Transplanted Heart

JEFFREY D. HOSENPUD AND MARK J. MORTON

There are substantial differences between the function of the cardiac allograft and the normal heart despite their similarities. Assessment of the transplanted heart and therapeutic intervention in transplant recipients require an understanding of these differences. This chapter will review the consequences of the transplant procedure on the transplanted heart and peripheral circulation, normal allograft function at rest and exercise, the response of the cardiac allograft to usual cardiovascular pharmacologic agents, and changes in cardiac function with rejection.

Cardiac Consequences of Transplantation

The heart continues to function satisfactorily after transplantation in most instances despite the many delicate mechanisms that have been disrupted by the nature of the procedure. Important considerations include mechanical effects related to attaching the atria, denervation, donor-recipient size matching, recipient hormonal milieu, and the immunologic consequences of rejection (Table 10.1).

Mechanical Considerations

Atrial booster pump function has been well characterized in normal and pathologic states in humans.[1,2] Normally, atrial systole contributes about 15% to 20% of the net stroke volume. This arrangement is disrupted by altering the pulse rate interval, ceasing atrial activity with stand-still or atrial fibrillation, or during retrograde atrial activation, which results in simultaneous atrial and ventricular systole. The atria in orthotopically transplanted hearts comprise roughly equal parts of donor and recipient atria. Without preexisting disease or surgical injury, the recipient sinoatrial (SA) node remains intact and paces the recipient atria at normal rates and with normal responses to physiologic and pharmacologic stimuli.[3,4] The suture lines act as an effective insulator, allowing the donor

TABLE 10.1. Factors potentially affecting cardiac function after transplantation.

Mechanical
    Reduced atrial booster pump function
    Donor-recipient size matching
    Preservation injury
    Denervation and denervation hypersensitivity
Recipient hormonal milieu
    Gender-specific hormones
    Renin-aldosterone
    Circulating catecholamines
    Atrial naturetic peptide
Rejection
    Myocytolysis
    Coronary vasculopathy
Immunosuppression
    Cyclosporine-induced hypertension
    Corticosteroid effects

and recipient atria to beat independently, although some tendency for isorhythmicity has been noted during exercise. The donor heart SA node is transplanted intact with its normal blood supply. Because the donor SA node is denervated, it beats at a rate close to the intrinsic rate and faster than the recipient sinus rate; thus, during most cardiac cycles the donor and recipient atria do not beat together, although the donor atrial-ventricular relationship remains normal (Fig. 10.1).

For these reasons, one would predict that the atrial booster pump function would be impaired after transplantation. To our knowledge, this has not been investigated rigorously. It has been our experience when studying patients by right and left heart catheterization that a waves, representing filling of the ventricles by the atrium, are smaller in some patients and not apparent in others after transplant. This finding supports the notion of reduced atrial booster pump function after transplantation.

It is unknown whether the effects of synchronization of the donor and recipient atria improve allograft hemodynamics. If this were the case, development of a pacing system that sensed the recipient's atrial rate (which

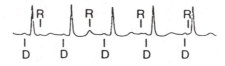

FIGURE 10.1. Electrocardiogram from a cardiac allograft recipient demonstrating both recipient (R) and donor (D) P waves. Note that the recipient P wave rate is slower and the P waves are not associated with the donor QRS complexes.

is more physiological) and then paced the donor atrium without delay might offer important hemodynamic advantages. However, the donor sinus node would need to be destroyed for this system to be effective.

Denervation

The effects of cardiac denervation in laboratory animals were reviewed by Donald in 1974.[5] The characteristic findings of denervation are increased, constant frequency of heart rate at rest, normal cardiac output, stroke volume, arterial pressure, LV dP/dt, and ejection rate. During exercise, heart rate increases slowly; with denervation increased cardiac output early in exercise depends more on the Starling mechanism than in normally innervated animals. Maximum capacity for exercise in denervated greyhounds is similar to sham-operated animals although performance is markedly blunted by administration of propranolol. The denervated heart responds normally to increases in blood pressure by maintaining stroke volume via the Starling mechanism, but rapid increases in cardiac output via heart rate, in response to reduced blood pressure, lag behind innervated hearts. Likewise, anemia or hypoxia produce smaller increases in cardiac output than for denervated animals because of the smaller increase in heart rate. Supersensitivity of the denervated heart to catecholamines is identified and is thought to compensate partially for the loss of direct innervation in this condition.

The recipient atrial cuff and pulmonary and systemic veins retain their innervation after human cardiac orthotopic transplantation. The donor SA node, atria, and ventricles are denervated by transection of the aorta, pulmonary artery, and atria. Reinnervation does not occur. Given the minimal resting chronotropic effect of the adrenergic nerves, resting donor sinus rate is increased because of vagal withdrawal. The resting heart rates in transplant recipients are similar to those noted by Jose and Taylor[6] after cardiac autonomic blockade with atropine and propranolol. Sinus node recovery time, AH, and HV intervals and response of the AV node to pacing are normal after transplantation. Atropine administration does not change donor rate but it does increase recipient rate.[7] These findings suggest that the major effect of the autonomic nervous system on cardiac conduction tissue at rest in the intact circulation is to decrease heart rate. Norepinephrine increases blood pressure, whereas isoproterenol results in vasodilation and a decrease in arterial pressure. Both agents increase donor sinus rate and decrease AH interval. Propranolol blocks the effects of isoproterenol and norepinephrine on donor rate and AH interval, but not the effect of norepinephrine on blood pressure.[8] Thus, donor heart rate after transplantation is affected primarily by circulating catecholamines.

The absence of vagal and adrenergic efferent innervation is most obvious in the lack of beat-to-beat heart rate control. Absence of cardiac afferent activity is more subtle. Thames et al.[9] showed that dogs with auto-transplanted hearts had increased blood volume and decreased renin responses to hemorrhage. Subsequently, Thames et al.[10] demonstrated in dogs that cardiopulmonary vagal afferents normally suppressed renin release. Furthermore, these receptors were more sensitive to blood volume changes than was the carotid baroreceptor. However, when cardiac denervation is performed, the carotid baroreceptors take over inhibition of renin release. Thus, cardiac vagal afferents may have an important role in the regulation of blood volume. In humans, Mohanty et al.[11] extended these findings to determine the significance of ventricular afferent denervation after cardiac transplantation. They showed that lower body negative pressure, an analog of hemorrhage, produced smaller increases in forearm vascular resistance and plasma norepinephrine levels in transplant recipients than normal controls. They excluded nonspecific causes by showing that the cold pressor test was normal in transplanted patients and that the lower body negative pressure response in renal transplant recipients who received an equal immunosuppressive regimen was normal. Thus, vagal afferent traffic sensitive to cardiac volume may be an important regulator of blood volume and arterial pressure, and these reflexes are abolished by transplantation.

We have noted one advantage to ventricular afferent denervation after transplantation. Normally, during injection of hypertonic radiocontrast material into the coronary arteries, sinus bradycardia and occasionally AV block and asystole can occur.[12] A dominant origin of this response is from afferent nerve stimulation, which results in vagal efferent output and bradycardia. Coronary angiography, which we perform routinely at yearly intervals or for evaluations of acute reductions in cardiac function, is remarkably free from radiocontrast-induced bradycardia in transplant recipients. Figure 10.2 shows a typical electrocardiogram and arterial pressure response to radiocontrast injection of renografin 76 in a normal patient and a patient 1 year after transplantation.

A final consequence of afferent denervation of the myocardium is the absence of ischemic myocardial pain. Thus, transplant recipients with severe vasculopathy and even infarction are usually pain-free. Transplant recipients with severe coronary disease or infarction may present with fatigue, congestive heart failure, syncope, or cardiogenic shock. Electrocardiographic changes typical for myocardial ischemia are unaltered by transplantation in this setting and should be sought. Evaluation of wall motion and coronary anatomy confirms the etiology of this picture. However, we recently studied a transplant recipient 2.5 years after grafting with a typical myocardial infarction syndrome. The location of his pain in the back, shoulders, and arms was unusual, but was heavy, oppressive, pressure-like discomfort. The electrocardiogram showed an anteroseptal infarction. Coronary and left ventriculography demonstrated left anterior descending artery occlusion, an anteroapical wall motion abnormality,

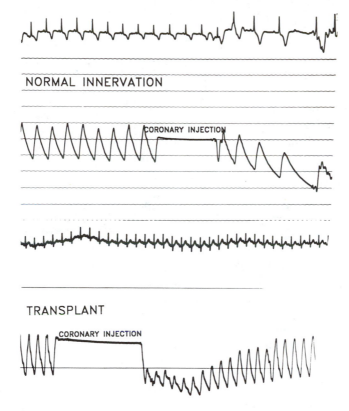

FIGURE 10.2. Heart rate and arterial pressure tracings from a normally innervated heart (top) and a cardiac allograft (bottom) after intracoronary contrast injection. Note the absence of bradycardia in the transplanted heart.

and advanced graft vasculopathy. We initially wondered if the patient's discomfort was related to ischemic pericarditis because the parietal pericardium is not resected and likely retains innervation. However, 2 weeks later the patient began having the identical pain on an intermittent basis that was relieved with nitroglycerine. The rapid progression of "silent" coronary artery disease provides the rationale for surveillance coronary angiography, which is performed yearly in most transplant programs.

The mechanisms for adrenergic hypersensitivity after cardiac transplantation in humans are now becoming understood. Hypersensitivity could be either presynaptic because of lack of catecholamine uptake by adrenergic neurons or postsynaptic because of changes in receptor density or second messenger activity. Gilbert et al.[13] offered strong evidence for a presynaptic origin. They showed that dose-response (heart rate) curves for isoproterenol were identical in donor and recipient atria, but left-shifted during epinephrine infusion in the donor atria. In addition,

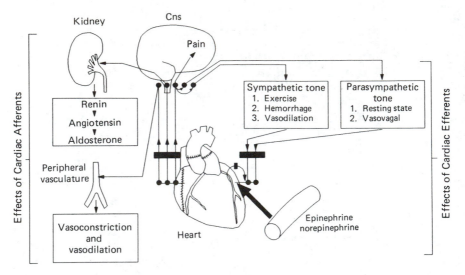

FIGURE 10.3. The effects of cardiac denervation involve the loss of both the cardiac afferents and efferents. The cardiac afferents have potential roles in salt and water regulation via the renin-angiotensin-aldosterone system, in reflex control of the peripheral vasculature, and in the sensation of cardiac pain. The cardiac efferents are responsible for the rapid changes in heart rate and contractility associated with changes in physiologic state. In addition, central reflexes are transmitted to the heart via the vagal efferent nerves. Finally, cardiac denervation results in hypersensitivity to circulating catecholamines caused by the lack of adrenergic neuronal transmittor uptake.

right ventricular endomyocardial biopsy samples had the same beta receptor densities as controls. These results differed from those of Yusuf et al.,[14] who found hypersensitivity to isoproterenol in the donor atrium. However, patients in the latter study were not pretreated with atropine and, thus, independent effects of vagal tone may be responsible for the disparate effects of isoproterenol on the innervated and denervated sinus nodes. Because epinephrine but not isoproterenol is normally taken up by the adrenergic nerves and because the adrenergic nerves are dead in transplanted hearts, supersensitivity to epinephrine is probably caused by a lack of uptake in the denervated hearts. Further support for this conclusion is drawn from the lack of an arteriovenous difference for catecholamines across the left ventricle in transplanted hearts. A summary of the effects of cardiac denervation are shown in Figure 10.3.

Hormonal Milieu

Little is known about the response of the transplanted heart to its new hormonal milieu. One important finding is the reversal of elevated cate-

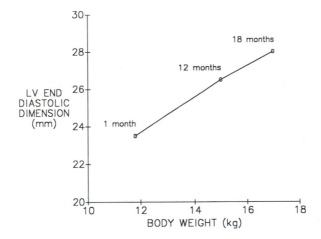

FIGURE 10.4. Left ventricular end-diastolic minor axis dimension as a function of recipient body weight in a patient transplanted at the age of 18 months. Note the gradual increase in heart size associated with the increase in body size over an 18-month period.

cholamines within several months after transplantation, a characteristic feature of patients with end-stage congestive heart failure.[15] The effects of transplanting male myocardium into females and vice versa are unknown. The possibility that myocardium is importantly affected by sex steroids is supported by experiments in animals[16] and during pregnancy and manipulation of hormone levels in humans.[17,18] Hearts transplanted in infants grow proportionally with the recipient body, but the mechanisms controlling cardiac growth in this setting are unknown (Fig. 10.4).

Resting Hemodynamics in Cardiac Allograft Recipients

Few studies have investigated allograft hemodynamics at specific time periods after cardiac transplantation. In fact, most have combined patients from multiple time periods, making interpretation of the data difficult. It is clear, however, that hemodynamics do change from the perioperative and very early postoperative periods to longer term after transplantation. Stinson and colleagues[20] investigated hemodynamics in 10 allograft recipients immediately postoperatively and for the first 7 days. Cardiac function was severely depressed immediately postoperatively (cardiac index: 1.8 L/min/m^2, stroke volume index: 21 ml/m^2) and then gradually improved over the subsequent 4 postoperative days to near normal. Isoproterenol provided significant improvement in stroke volume index in the six patients who were treated, with their cardiac index increasing even more substantially because of the associated increase in

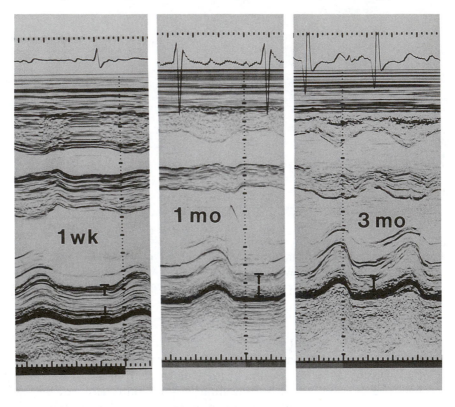

FIGURE 10.5. Serial echocardiograms from a patient after cardiac transplantation demonstrating the progressive decrease in wall thickness over time. Reproduced from Hosenpud et al. (1987),[22] with permission.

heart rate. These data provide the basis for the routine use of isoproterenol immediately after transplantation.

Two studies have investigated allograft function within the first week and compared this to late allograft function. Davies and colleagues demonstrated that allograft ejection fractions were stable between study dates; however, filling pressures were significantly elevated early posttransplantation and normalized over time. The elevation in filling pressures was not correlated with the presence of rejection.[21] Work from our program expanded on these data by comparing echocardiographic findings at 1 week and 1 and 3 months posttransplantation.[22] As with the previous study, filling pressures were initially high but subsequently normalized. In addition, left ventricular wall thickness and calculated left ventricular myocardial volume was substantially increased over normal levels, presumably secondary to myocardial edema, but gradually normalized over the 3-month period. Figure 10.5 demonstrates the M-mode echocardiogram from one patient showing a progressive reduction in left

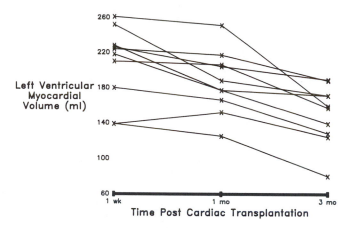

FIGURE 10.6. Calculated myocardial volumes in 10 patients after cardiac transplantation demonstrating a serial decline in myocardial volume (mass), from 1 week to 3 months. Reproduced from Hosenpud et al. (1987),[22] with permission.

ventricular wall thickness. Figure 10.6 demonstrates the calculated myocardial volumes for the study group, again demonstrating the gradual fall in myocardial volume (mass). We speculate that these volume changes represent edema from preservation injury. Furthermore, the sequential improvement in allograft systolic and diastolic function after transplantation may be importantly related to the reduction of edema.

The most obvious alteration in hemodynamics of allograft recipients is the increased heart rate. This occurs because of the loss of resting vagal tone, which normally suppresses the intrinsic heart rate. In contrast to the normal heart rate of approximately 70 beats per min (bpm),[23] resting allograft heart rates in our patient population are 93 ± 11 bpm (n = 55) at 3 months and 90 ± 11 bpm (n = 38) at 1 year, with ranges of 72 bpm to 115 bpm. Several studies (including our own) have demonstrated that stable allograft right and left heart filling pressures are either at the upper limits of normal levels or slightly increased.[22,24–28] Cardiac outputs (indices) are reported either as normal or at the lower limits of normal.[25–28] Of some interest are the smaller than normal indexed left ventricular end-diastolic volumes and, hence, stroke volumes consistently reported[28–30] but currently unexplained. Possible explanations might include rejection and scar formation, to date an unexplained effect of immunosuppression, or the chronic elevation in heart rate. Although the first two explanations are feasible, patients with no history of rejection also tend to have small hearts, and the reduced volumes were reported before the use of cyclosporine, thereby eliminating that agent as a potential candidate. Although data investigating the effects on the left ventricle of a chronically elevated heart rate are not available, the dilatory response of the left ventricle to a chronically reduced heart rate is well described.[31]

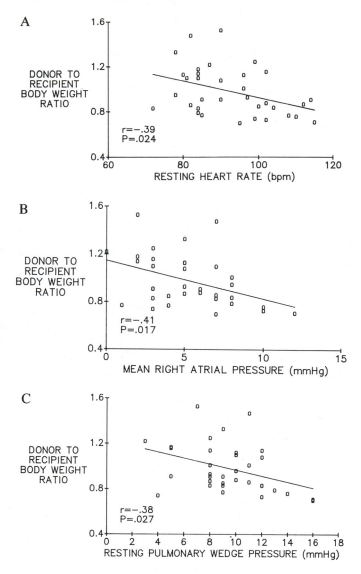

FIGURE 10.7. Three months after cardiac transplantation there is a negative correlation between the donor:recipient body weight ratio and heart rate (A), right atrial (B) and pulmonary wedge pressures (C), respectively, in 34 patients. This would suggest that relatively smaller hearts require increased heart rates and filling pressures to maintain cardiac output. Reproduced from Hosenpud et al. (1989),[34] with permission.

There have been at least two reports suggesting that the cardiac allograft develops myocardial restriction over time, possibly secondary to rejection or cyclosporine administration.[32,33] This scenario would potentially explain the mild elevation in filling pressures, reduced cardiac volumes, and low normal or reduced cardiac outputs previously discussed. Studies from our institution suggest another explanation for the apparent "restrictive" physiology.[34] The cardiac transplant circulation is unique because the heart is only marginally matched in size to the body. Most centers use a weight range of ±20% (some centers up to 30%), to match donors and recipients. No real accounting is made for differences in body habitus, age, and myocardial mass differences associated with sex.[35] The assumption is that the heart will ultimately adapt to the recipient body size. If this is not the case, those receiving relatively small hearts would tend to be "restricted" and those receiving relatively larger hearts would tend to have low filling pressures. Figure 10.7 demonstrates the statistically significant negative correlations between the donor/recipient body weight ratio and heart rates, right atrial pressures and pulmonary wedge pressures, respectively, in 34 patients 3 months after cardiac transplantation. These data would strongly support the above hypothesis that the donor heart fails to adapt to the recipient body before 3 months after cardiac transplantation. Those with smaller hearts require higher heart rates and filling pressures to maintain adequate cardiac output. The impact of chronic elevations in heart rate and filling pressures on ultimate cardiac function might not be favorable.

Exercise Hemodynamics after Cardiac Transplantation

As previously noted, in the normally innervated heart, heart rate at rest is substantially lower than for transplanted hearts.[23] During isotonic exercise, heart rate in normal hearts increases promptly and in proportion to the amount of work. The increment in cardiac output during supine exercise is primarily caused by increased heart rate; stroke volume plays only a minor role in most studies.[23,29,36] The mechanism by which stroke volume is increased during supine isotonic exercise is a reduction in end-systolic volume caused by increased contractility and decreased afterload.[23,26,37]

Left ventricular filling pressure does increases slightly during supine exercise in normal hearts.[23] It appears that in normal supine individuals, the heart is operating at or near the "break point" of the function curve and uses preload minimally, if at all, to increase cardiac output.[29,36,37] This is in contrast to upright exercise, where both heart rate and stroke volume are used for increasing cardiac output.[38] The increase in stroke volume is accompanied by an increase in filling pressures over resting levels (although still within the normal range), presumably mediated by the transport of blood volume centrally via the peripheral muscle pump.[23] This

TABLE 10.2. Rest and exercise pressures and flows one year after cardiac transplantation.

Parameter	Normal[a]	Rest	Exercise
Right atrial (mmHg)	0–8	6 ± 2	14 ± 7
Pulmonary artery mean (mmHg)	9–16	18 ± 3	32 ± 9
Pulmonary wedge (mmHg)	1–10	10 ± 3	20 ± 6
Cardiac output (L/min)	—	5.0 ± .9	9.9 ± 1.7
Cardiac index (L/min/m²)	2.8–4.2	2.5 ± .5	5.0 ± .8
Stroke volume (ml)	—	55 ± 9	77 ± 13
Stroke volume index (ml/m²)	30–56	28 ± 6	39 ± 7
Heart rate (bpm)	—	90 ± 11	122 ± 18
Mean arterial pressure (mmHg)	70–105	91 ± 12	102 ± 14
SVR (Wood units)	10–19	17.7 ± 4.0	9.3 ± 2.4

[a]Data from Grossman WH,[41] Cardiac Catheterization and Angiography, Lea & Febiger, Philadelphia, 1986.

would suggest that in normal upright individuals, the heart is operating much lower on the function curve.

To date, the hemodynamic assessment of the transplanted human heart has been performed exclusively in the supine position. Differences with the normally innervated heart therefore will be discussed with this in mind. It is clear that the denervated heart contributes to the exercise response using different mechanisms compared to a normally innervated heart. As early as 1970, Campeau and colleagues demonstrated a reduced heart rate response to supine isotonic exercise associated with a dramatic increase in left ventricular end-diastolic pressure in transplant patients.[24] They interpreted these findings as evidence for myocardial dysfunction perhaps related to chronic rejection or catecholamine depletion secondary to the denervated state.

Alternative explanations were provided by Stinson and colleagues, who defined the exercise response in patients 1 and 2 years after cardiac transplantation.[39] They demonstrated elevated resting heart rates, a very gradual increase in heart rate with exercise, a rapid increase in left ventricular end-diastolic pressure, and a substantial increase in cardiac output owing to an increase in stroke volume. Thus, the transplanted heart relied heavily on the Frank-Starling mechanism for increased cardiac output because of a much attenuated heart rate response, especially early after the onset of exercise. Later, the Stanford group measured end-diastolic volume directly at rest, during volume loading (leg lifting), and with graded supine bicycle exercise.[40] As predicted, end-diastolic volume increased along with end-diastolic pressure, confirming the role of the Frank-Starling mechanism at least for early exercise. This finding has been substantiated more recently using radionuclide ventriculography by studies from our program[28] and others.[29]

Table 10.2 demonstrates supine rest and bicycle exercise right atrial

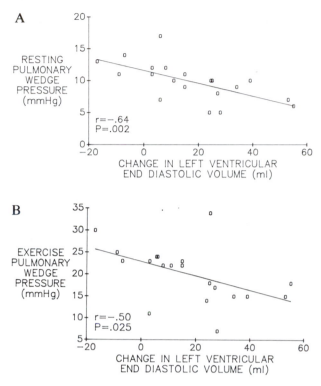

FIGURE 10.8. One year after cardiac transplantation, there is a negative correlation between the change in left ventricular end-diastolic volume from rest (A) to exercise (B) and resting and exercise pulmonary wedge pressures, respectively. Therefore, those patients with the ability to increase preload (sarcomere length) with exercise have lower filling pressures. Reproduced from Hosenpud et al. (1989),[28] with permission.

and pulmonary wedge pressures in 23 allograft recipients 1 year after cardiac transplantation. The most notable findings are the striking elevations in ventricular filling pressures and the subtantial increase in stroke volume with exercise. Figure 10.8 demonstrates statistically significant negative correlations between the change in left ventricular end-diastolic volume with exercise and the resting and exercise pulmonary wedge pressures, respectively. This inverse relationship between rest and exercise left ventricular filling pressures and the ability to increase left ventricular end-diastolic volume with exercise suggests that some cardiac transplant recipients are not operating on the "break point" of the left ventricular function curve but may be anywhere along it. Normal individuals operate near the "break point" (Figure 10.9 point #1 top and bottom). At this point, a small increase in left ventricular volume causes a substantial increase in filling pressure as intravascular volume is shunted

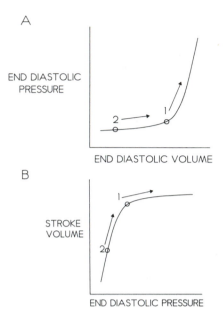

FIGURE 10.9. A, Schematic showing the normal left ventricular diastolic pressure-volume relation. B, Schematic showing the normal left ventricular function curve. Patient 1 is operating at or above optimal filling pressures at rest. With exercise (arrow), there is little or no gain in filling volume or resultant stroke volume with a substantial increase in filling pressure. Patient 2 is operating below optimal filling pressures at rest. With the onset of exercise, filling pressures increase only modestly with the increase in left ventricular volume and stroke volume (preload reserve). Reproduced from Hosenpud et al. (1989),[28] with permission.

centrally with the onset of exercise. Little increase in stroke volume results. Cardiac transplant recipients who receive relatively smaller hearts might be operating at or beyond point #1. Recipients receiving relatively larger hearts, presumably with "preload reserve", may be operating on the ascending limb of the function curve (Figure 10.9, point #2 top and bottom), where a larger increase in left ventricular volume causes a smaller increase in left ventricular filling pressure and a larger increase in stroke volume. These findings are consistent with prior observations that preload reserve or end-diastolic volume is used to augment cardiac output during supine exercise in patients after cardiac transplantation.[29] Although the increased end-diastolic volume and increased ejection fraction effectively increases exercise stroke volume, the higher than normal filling pressures reach levels that may produce symptoms of dyspnea and cause a reduction in exercise capacity.

Only one study has investigated the cardiovascular response to isometric exercise after cardiac transplantation. Savin and colleagues[42] measured heart rate, blood pressure, and left ventricular volumes at rest and during 50% maximal voluntary handgrip in patients after transplantation and compared them to patients with innervated hearts. Arterial pressure increased similarly in both groups, consistent with an intact peripheral circulatory response to isometric exercise. Heart rate did not change in the transplant group, but, as expected, it increased in patients with normal cardiac innervation. End-diastolic volume increased only in the transplant patients, resulting in an increase in stroke volume, despite an ejection fraction that fell slightly. The net result was an increase in cardiac output similar in magnitude to that found in the innervated patients. Therefore, the denervated heart is highly dependent on preload for an adequate response to exercise, whether the exercise is isometric or isotonic.

Allograft Response to Cardiac Drugs

The actions of drugs in the transplant recipient can be predicted from the knowledge of the physiology of denervation:

1. Reflex cardiac stimulation by adrenergic or parasympathetic nerves will not occur.
2. The cardiac response to epinephrine and norepinephrine will be enhanced because of supersensitivity.
3. The cardiac response to adrenergic antagonists will be enhanced because of the reliance on circulating catecholamines.
4. Drugs that stimulate cardiac afferents will have no effect.

Several examples of drug effects in transplant recipients are listed in Table 10.3. The most important example of absent reflex stimulation occurs with administration of digitalis. Whereas the inotropic action of digitalis probably directly affects the myocardium, the most important clinical action of this drug as an antiarrhythmic agent is the reflex stimulation of the vagus nerve. The putative mechanism for this effect is sensitization of the carotid sinus baroreceptor; thus, Goodman et al.[43] found no effect of acute intravenous digitalization in transplant recipients on atrial effective refractory period, functional refractory period, AV node effective refractory period, functional refractory period, or response to pacing. In contrast, digitalization in normal subjects produced prolongation of the AV node effective and functional refractory periods. Accordingly, digitalization to slow the ventricular response in atrial fibrillation or flutter is useless after transplantation. Verapamil, which acts directly on the slow-calcium channel in the AV node, slows AV conduction equally well in transplanted and nontransplanted hearts. Conversely, quinidine, which

TABLE 10.3. Cardiovascular drugs after cardiac transplantation.

Drug	Effect in recipient	Mechanism
Digitalis	Normal increase in contractility, minimal AV nodal effect	Denervation
Atropine	None	Denervation
Epinephrine	Increased contractility and chronotropy	Denervation hypersensitivity
Norepinephrine	Increased contractility and chronotropy	Denervation hypersensitivity
Isoproterenol	Normal increase in inotropy and chronotropy	No neuronal uptake
Quinidine	No vagalytic effect	Denervation
Verapamil	Normal AV block	Direct effect
Nifedipine	No reflex tachycardia	Denervation
Hydralazine	No reflex tachycardia	Denervation
Beta blockers	Increased antagonist effect during exercise	Denervation

may have a vagalytic effect, should not be given without adequate digitalization to normally innervated patients with atrial fibrillation or flutter, but can be given without concern for accelerating AV conduction to transplant recipients with these arrhythmias.

Another important example is the lack of reflex tachycardia associated with administration of vasodilating agents. This phenomenon is beneficial when hypertension is being treated with hydralazine or nifedipine. In the intact circulation, use of either of these agents usually requires concomitant beta blocker therapy, which is unnecessary after cardiac transplantation. Conversely, the lack of homeostatic, rapid adjustments in heart rate to sudden drug-induced changes in vascular resistance can produce wide swings in blood pressure. The latter effect can be particularly troublesome during anesthesia.

Changes in Allograft Function with Acute Rejection

Signs and symptoms of left ventricular systolic dysfunction were commonly associated with cardiac allograft rejection in the precyclosporine era.[44–46] With the institution of surveillance endomyocardial biopsy and cyclosporine immunosuppression, systolic allograft dysfunction by most reports[47–49] and our own experience is a late phenomenon and in many cases is a premorbid event. Because of the insensitivity of ejection phase indicies of systolic cardiac function, many studies have investigated diastole as a potentially more sensitive measure of allograft function and hence a possible marker for allograft rejection. Dawkins and colleagues demonstrated that the mean isovolumic relaxation period, assessed by echocardiography, fell with progressive rejection severity.[47] The authors interpreted these findings to suggest that left atrial pressure increases secondary to reduced ventricular compliance, causing early mitral valve closure. These findings were subsequently confirmed by Haverich et al.[48] and Desruennes et al.[49] Paulsen and colleagues demonstrated a prolonged rapid filling period with rejection.[50] In most of these studies, the overlap of diastolic indicies between patients with and without rejection was substantial, making their clinical usefulness, at the current time, still a matter for investigation. However, it is clear from these studies that changes in left ventricular diastolic function occur early and to variable degrees with allograft rejection.

Recommendations for the Cardiac Allograft Recipient

Based on the physiology of the cardiac allograft and its new circulation, one can draw certain conclusions and make recommendations for activity in patients after transplantation. Given the substantial dependence on preload, it would be anticipated that those patients with the largest preload reserve would likely be most able to exercise successfully. Based on studies from our institution, the optimal way to accomplish this is to oversize the donor heart with respect to the recipient. Unfortunately, given the shortage of donor organs and the instability of the patient population, this is not possible in most cases.

Without significant preload reserve, patients after cardiac transplantation depend even more on circulating catecholamines to increase heart rate and contractility in order to increase cardiac output during exercise. A warm-up period (between 5 and 10 min of activity) before strenuous exercise is therefore mandatory. In addition, although beta blocking agents can be tried cautiously in low dosages after transplantation, they can produce significant exercise impairment in some patients.

Because of the inadequate heart rate response to hypotension, postural changes in blood pressure will be more pronounced, especially when there has been significant periods of inactivity (prolonged bed rest) or situations associated with cutaneous vasodilation (sun bathing, hot tubs, etc.). In these instances, care should be taken to shift gradually from supine to the upright position. For the same reasons, medications that alter systemic vascular resistance should be used cautiously. This would include antihypertensives, which produce direct arterial vasodilation and especially anesthesia. In patients requiring surgery with either general or spinal anesthesia, one must be prepared to use arterial vasocontricting agents to prevent potentially serious hypotension during induction. In some instances, a test dose of an alpha agent (ephedrine or phenylephrine) has been helpful to determine dose responsiveness in a given patient before the induction of general or spinal anesthesia.

Conclusions

The cardiovascular system is altered dramatically after cardiac transplantation. The issues of cardiac denervation, size matching, hormonal milieu, drug effects, and rejection all need to be considered when evaluating and advising patients after cardiac transplantation. In addition to specific transplantation issues, cardiac transplantation provides a unique model for understanding cardiovascular adaptation in general.

References

1. Rahimtoola SH, Ehsani A, Sinno MZ, et al. Left atrial transport function in myocardial infarction: importance of its booster pump function. *Am J Med.* 1975;59:686–694.
2. Stott DK, Marpole DGF, Bristow JD, et al. The role of left atrial transport in aortic and mitral stenosis. *Circulation.* 1970;41:1031–1041.
3. Leachman RD, Cokkinos DVP, Zamalloa O, et al. Electrocardiographic behavior of recipient and donor atria after human heart transplantation. *Am J Cardiol.* 1969;24:49–53.
4. Stinson EB, Schroeder JS, Griepp RB, et al. Observations on the behavior of recipient atria after cardiac transplantation in man. *Am J Cardiol.* 1972;30:615–622.
5. Donald DE. Myocardial performance after excision of the extrinsic cardiac nerves in the dog. *Circ Res.* 1974;34:417–424.
6. Jose AD, Taylor RR. Autonomic blockade by propranolol and atropine to study intrinsic myocardial function in man. *J Clin Invest.* 1969;48:2019–2031.
7. Cannom DS, Graham AF, Harrison DL. Electrophysiological studies in the denervated transplanted human heart: response to atrial pacing and atropine. *Circ Res.* 1973;32:268–278.
8. Cannom DS, Rider AK, Stinson EB, et al. Electrophysiologic studies in the denervated transplanted human heart. II. Response to norepinephrine, isoproterenol and propranolol. *Am J Cardiol.* 1975;36:859–866.
9. Thames MD, Hassan ZU, Brackett NC, et al. Plasma renin responses to hemorrhage after cardiac autotransplantation. *Am J Physiol.* 1971;221:1115–1119.
10. Thames MD, Jarecki M, Donald DE. Neural control of renin secretion in anesthetized dogs: interaction of cardiopulmonary and carotid baroreceptors. *Circ Res.* 1978;42:237–245.
11. Mohanty PK, Thames MD, Arrowood JA, Sowers JE, McNamara C, Szentpetery S. Impairment of cardiopulmonary baroreflex after cardiac transplantation in humans. *Circulation.* 1987;75:914–921.
12. Larsen GC, Hosenpud JD. Pharmacologic and anaphylactoid reactions to radiocontrast media. In: Kron J, Morton MJ, eds. *Complications of Cardiac Catheterization and Angiography: Prevention and Management.* Mount Kisco, NY: Futura Publishing Co; 1989:239–267.
13. Gilbert EM, Eiswirth CC, Mealey PC, et al. β-Adrenergic supersensitivity of the transplanted human heart is presynaptic in origin. *Circulation.* 1989;79:344–349.

14. Yusuf S, Theodoropoulos S, Mathias CJ, et al. Increased sensitivity of the denervated transplanted human heart to isoprenaline both before and after β-adrenergic blockade. *Circulation*. 1987;75:696–704.

15. Olivari MT, Levine TB, Ring WS, et al. Normalization of sympathetic nervous system function after orthotopic cardiac transplant in man. *Circulation*. 1987;76(suppl V):V62–V64.

16. Scheuer J, Malhotra A, Schaible TF, et al. Effects of gonadectomy and hormonal replacement on rat hearts. *Circ Res*. 1987;61:12–19.

17. Robson SC, Hunter S, Boys RJ, et al. Serial study of factors influencing changes in cardiac output during human pregnancy. *Am J Physiol*. 1989;256:H1060–H1065.

18. Veille JC, Morton MJ, Burry K, et al. Estradiol and hemodynamics during ovulation induction. *J Clin Endocrin Metab*. 1986;63:721–724.

19. Donald DE, Shepherd JT. Reflexes from the heart and lungs: physiological curiosities or important regulatory mechanisms. *Cardiovasc Res*. 1978;12:449–469.

20. Stinson EB, Caves PK, Griepp RB, Oyer PE, Rider AK, Shumway NE. Hemodynamic observations in the early period after human heart transplantation. *J Thorac Cardiovasc Surg*. 1975;69:264–270.

21. Davies RA, Koshal A, Walley V, et al. Temporary diastolic noncompliance with preserved systolic function after heart transplantation. *Transplant Proc*. 1987;19:3444–3447.

22. Hosenpud JD, Norman DJ, Cobanoglu MA, Floten HS, Conner RM, Starr A. Serial echocardiographic findings early after heart transplantation: evidence for reversible right ventricular dysfunction and myocardial edema. *J Heart Transplant*. 1987;6:343–347.

23. Thadani U, Parker JO. Hemodynamics at rest and during supine and sitting bicycle exercise in normal subjects. *Am J Cardiol*. 1978;41:52–59.

24. Campeau L, Pospisil L, Grondin P, Dyrda I, Lepage G. Cardiac catheterization findings at rest and after exercise in patients following cardiac transplantation. *Am J Cardiol*. 1970;25:523–528.

25. Pflugfelder PW, McKenzie FN, Kostuk WJ. Hemodynamic profiles at rest and during supine exercise after orthotopic cardiac transplantation. *Am J Cardiol*. 1988;61:1328–1333.

26. Greenberg ML, Uretsky BF, Reddy PS, et al. Long-term hemodynamic follow-up of cardiac transplant patients treated with cyclosporine and prednisone. *Circulation*. 1985;71:487–494.

27. Hosenpud JD, Pantely GA, Morton MJ, et al. Lack of progressive "restrictive" physiology following transplantation despite intervening episodes of allograft rejection: a comparison of serial rest and exercise hemodynamics one and two years post transplantation. *J Heart Transplant*. 1989;8:241–244.

28. Hosenpud JD, Morton MJ, Wilson RA, et al. Abnormal exercise hemodynamics in cardiac allograft recipients one year following cardiac transplantation: relationship to preload reserve. *Circulation*. 1989;80:525–532.

29. Pflugfelder PW, Purves PD, McKenzie FN, Kostuk WJ: Cardiac dynamics during supine exercise in cyclosporine-treated orthotopic heart transplant recipients: assessment by radionuclide angiography. *J Am Coll Cardiol*. 1987;10:336–341.

30. Borow KM, Neumann A, Arensman FW, Yacoub MH. Left ventricular con-

tractility and contractile reserve in humans after cardiac transplantation. *Circulation*. 1985;71:866–872.

31. Starzl TE, Gaertner RA: Chronic heart block in dogs. A method for producing experimental heart failure. *Circulation*. 1955;12:259–271.

32. Humen DP, McKenzie FN, Kostuk WJ. Restricted myocardial compliance one year following cardiac transplantation. *J Heart Transplant*. 1984;3:341–345.

33. Young JB, Leon CA, Short D III, et al. Evolution of hemodynamics after orthotopic heart and heart-lung transplantation: early restrictive patterns persisting in an occult fashion. *J Heart Transplant*. 1987;6:34–43.

34. Hosenpud JD, Pantely GA, Morton MJ, Norman DJ, Cobanoglu AM, Starr A. Relationship between recipient:donor body size matching and hemodynamics 3 months following cardiac transplantation. *J Heart Transplant*. 1989;8:241–243.

35. Kennedy JW, Baxley WA, Figley MM, Dodge HT, Blackmon JR. Quantitative angiocardiography. I. The normal left ventricle in man. *Circulation*. 1966;34:272–278.

36. Ross J, Linhart JW, Braunwald E. Effects of changing heart rate in man by electrical stimulation of the right atrium. Studies at rest, during exercise and with isoproterenol. *Circulation*. 1965;32:549–58.

37. Parker JO, Case RB. Normal left ventricular function. *Circulation*. 1979;60:4–12.

38. Crawford MH, White DH, Amon KW. Echocardiographic evaluation of left ventricular size and performance during handgrip and supine and upright bicycle exercise. *Circulation*. 1979;59:1188–1196.

39. Stinson EB, Griepp RB, Schroeder JS, Dong E Jr, Shumway NE. Hemodynamic observations one and two years after cardiac transplantation in man. *Circulation*. 1972;45:1183–1193.

40. Pope SE, Stinson EB, Daughters GT, Schroeder JS, Ingels NB, Alderman EL. Exercise response of the denervated heart in long-term cardiac transplant recipients. *Am J Cardiol*. 1980;46:213–218

41. Grossman WH. *Cardiac Catheterization and Angiography*. Philadelphia, Penn: Lea & Febiger; 1986.

42. Savin WM, Alderman EL, Haskell WL, Schroeder JS, Ingels NB Jr, Daughters GT. Left ventricular response to isometric exercise in patients with denervated and innervated hearts. *Circulation*. 1980;61:897–901.

43. Goodman DJ, Rossen RM, Cannom DS, et al. Effect of digoxin on atrioventricular conduction: studies in patients with and without cardiac autonomic innervation. *Circulation*. 1975;51:251–256.

44. Griepp RB, Stinson EB, Dong E Jr, Clark DA, Shumway NE. Acute rejection of the allografted human heart. *Ann Thorac Surg*. 1971;12:113–126.

45. Leachman RD, Cokkinos DVP, Rochelle DG, et al. Serial hemodynamic study of the transplanted heart and correlation with clinical rejection. *J Thorac Cardiovasc Surg*. 1971;61:561–569.

46. Stinson EB, Tecklenberg PL, Hollingsworth JF, Jones KW, Sloane R, Rahmoeller G. Changes in left ventricular mechanical and hemodynamic function during acute rejection of orthotopically transplanted hearts in dogs. *J Cardiovasc Surg*. 1974;68:783–791.

47. Dawkins KD, Oldershaw PJ, Billingham ME, et al. Changes in diastolic function as a noninvasive marker of cardiac allograft rejection. *J Heart Transplant*. 1984;3:286–294.
48. Haverich A, Kemnitz J, Fieguth HG, et al. Non-invasive parameters for detection of cardiac allograft rejection. *Clin Transplant*. 1987;1:151–158.
49. Desruennes M, Corcos T, Cabrol A, et al. Doppler echocardiolgraphy for the diagnosis of acute cardiac allograft rejection. *J Am Coll Cardiol*. 1988;12:63–70.
50. Paulsen W, Magid N, Sagar K, et al. Left ventricular function of heart allografts during acute rejection: an echocardiographic assessment. *J Heart Transplant*. 1985;4:525–529.

11
Medical Complications in Patients after Cardiac Transplantation

JOHN B. O'CONNELL

Although cardiologists and cardiac surgeons commonly serve as the primary care physicians for cardiac transplant recipients, the complications that develop may transcend their specific area of expertise and training.[1] Despite the functional differences between the denervated allograft and the normal heart, severe cardiac dysfunction is distinctly unusual.[2] The medical complications that follow cardiac transplantation involve multiple organ systems and require the input of specialists in such broad areas as infectious diseases, nephrology, gastroenterology, neurology, endocrinology, gynecology, pulmonology, and oncology. Therefore, the physician who is primarily responsible for the patient's care must assume the role of a generalist and recruit the support of the appropriate specialists when necessary.

The major life-threatening complication after cardiac transplantation is allograft rejection. Appropriately, the primary emphasis of research during the initial clinical application was establishing effective immunosuppressive regimens.[3] The use of routine surveillance endomyocardial biopsy and prompt intervention with potent immunosuppression have decreased the mortality caused by rejection. However, the complications of immunosuppressive therapy have now become a major source of medical morbidity (Table 11.1). The purpose of this chapter is to review the medical complications after cardiac transplantation.

Infection

Immunosuppression attenuates the host response to infection particularly when intensification is required for the treatment of allograft rejection. As a result, infection has become the most common cause of death after cardiac transplantation.[4] In the precyclosporine era, the number of infections rose from 1.3 to 3.6 per 1000 patient days after intensification of immunosuppression for the treatment of allograft rejection.[5] After the introduction of cyclosporine, a more potent and selective immunosuppres-

TABLE 11.1. Common medical complications after cardiac transplantation.

Attributed to immunosuppression
  Infection
  Hypertension
  Gastrointestinal lesions
    Esophagitis, ulcers, diverticulitis, ileus, hepatitis, cholelithiasis, pancreatitis
  Renal dysfunction
  Endocrine/metabolic complications
    Diabetes mellitus, osteoporosis, osteonecrosis, growth retardation, reproductive
      dysfunction, hyperlipidemia
  Seizures
  Malignancy
Independent of immunosuppression
  Cardiac allograft vasculopathy

sive agent, the incidence of infection causing death has decreased, possibly owing to a reduction in corticosteroid usage. Hofflin et al. compared patients receiving prednisone, azathioprine, and rabbit antithymocyte globulin to those receiving cyclosporine and prednisone and found that infection lead to death in 39% of the control patients and 11% of the cyclosporine group.[6] Dresdale et al. reported that 55% of patients never experienced an infection when even lower dosages of cyclosporine and prednisone were used.[7] Routine use of cyclosporine has resulted not only in a total reduction of infections, but more importantly in a profound decrease in bacterial infections. In a recent survey of 655 recipients in 24 heart transplant centers, there were 0.66 episodes of infection per recipient.[8] Forty-five percent of the infections were viral, only 34% bacterial, 9% fungal, and 8% protozoal compared to 84% of all infections caused by bacteria in the precyclosporine era.[5]

Surgical complications remain the primary source of purulent bacterial infections, which include mediastinitis, pneumonia, urinary tract infections, and intravenous catheter-related sepsis. Mediastinitis is a serious complication that requires prolonged therapy with intravenous antibiotics and adequate drainage by mediastinal exploration with irrigation, followed by surgery for sternal closure and/or repair using skeletal muscle flaps.[9,10] Perioperative purulent bacterial infections are best prevented by sterile technique for insertion and early discontinuation of chest tubes, intravenous lines, and bladder catheters. Aggressive respiratory therapy focused toward improving postoperative atelectasis is a useful adjunct in the prevention of bacterial pneumonias. These early complications are common to all cardiac surgery and close attention to detail can minimize the frequency.

Infections in cardiac transplant patients are frequently caused by opportunistic organisms that induce serious illness only in the immunocompromised host (Table 11.2). Transmission of opportunistic infections by the donor organ and blood products can be minimized but not totally

TABLE 11.2. Opportunistic
infections after cardiac
transplantation.

Donor organ/blood product transmission
  CMV
  Toxoplasma gondii
  HIV
Air, water, or fecal transmission
  Legionella pneumophilia
  Pneumocytis carinii
  Listeria monocytogenes
  Nocardia asteroides
  Aspergillus sp.
  Candida sp.

avoided.[11] Organisms transmitted by this mechanism include cytomegalovirus (CMV), human immunodeficiency virus (HIV), and *Toxoplasma
gondii*. Other sources of infection include latent viruses such as Herpes
simplex and herpes zoster that reactivate with intensive immunosuppression. Air, water, and fecal-borne organisms that result in serious illness
in immunocompromised hosts include *Legionella pneumophila, Pneumocystis carinii, Listeria monocytogenes,* and *Nocardia asteroides*. It has
been proposed that reverse isolation may minimize exposure to these organisms. However, recent analysis of the effect of protective isolation on
infection rate after cardiac transplantation showed no difference between
patients who were protected by private room, hat, sterile gown, hand
washing, and mask compared with those who were treated with standard
infection control measures and hand washing.[12]

Cytomegalovirus

Cytomegalovirus is the most common infection transmitted by the donor
organ. Fifty percent to 80% of adults have detectable antibodies to CMV
in the peripheral blood. If the recipient is CMV-seronegative and receives
a heart from a seropositive donor, there is a strong likelihood that CMV
will be transmitted. Although it is possible to transplant CMV-seronegative donors selectively into CMV-seronegative recipients, it is frequently
not practical to restrict the transplantation of the donor heart into a critically ill recipient based solely on CMV antibody status.

Although the role of blood transfusions in transmitting CMV is not well
defined, most heart transplant centers have tried to avoid this possibility
by using blood from CMV-negative donors or by washing or filtering
blood to remove leukocytes that can harbor the virus. A primary CMV
infection (occurring in a seronegative recipient receiving a heart from a
seropositive donor) can result in pronounced symptomatic disease that is

TABLE 11.3. Characteristics of cytomegalovirus infection.

Presentation
    Illness more severe in primary infection compared to reactivation
    May be systemic or localized to lungs, retina, gastrointestinal tract, or liver
Treatment
    Ganciclovir (DHPG) 20 mg/kg/day IV for 10–14 days
    Hyperimmune CMV or pooled gamma globulin
Prevention
    Avoid seropositive blood products and organs in CMV-seronegative
      recipients
    Acyclovir 800–3200 mg po
    Hyperimmune CMV or pooled gamma globulin

more severe than reactivation of endogenous CMV caused by immuno-suppression.[13] However, since CMV has multiple serotypes, a de novo primary infection can rarely occur in a CMV-seropositive recipient.[14]

The clinical manifestations of CMV infection are protean (Table 11.3). The infection may be asymptomatic, manifested only by seroconversion (a four-fold rise of antibody titer within 4 to 8 weeks of transplantation). When symptomatic, the systemic manifestations of infection include fever, malaise, and anorexia. If the infection localizes to the lungs, gastrointestinal tract, or retina, serious, life-threatening disease may result. Cytomegalovirus infection is a common cause of interstitial pneumonia with fever and hypoxia.[15] Because the virus may be shed in the bronchial secretions without clinical pneumonia, nuclear inclusions in cells obtained by bronchoalveolar lavage must be identified before the diagnosis can be confirmed. The gastrointestinal manifestations of CMV infection include ulcers at any location in the gut. When endoscopy demonstrates ulcerations, culture of washings or biopsy must be obtained to establish the diagnosis. Cytomegalovirus is a cause of hepatitis that rarely will be confused with cyclosporine or azathioprine hepatotoxicity, which more commonly are cholestatic. Cytomegalovirus chorioretinitis and papillitis results in visual loss.[16] A careful retinal examination must be performed in patients who have fever and visual loss. A rare manifestation of CMV infection is myocarditis, which may result in cardiac dysfunction and must be differentiated from allograft rejection.[17]

When a transplant recipient has unexplained fever in the first 12 weeks after surgery, cultures of the urine and peripheral blood buffy coat may identify CMV replication. If the virus has localized to the lungs or gastrointestinal tract, an aggressive invasive diagnostic evaluation should be pursued. Treatment with ganciclovir should be considered when CMV localizes to a specific organ.[18,19] Ganciclovir, a guanine analogue, inhibits viral-induced deoxyribonucleic acid (DNA) polymerase and prevents viral replication. In life-threatening illness, CMV-specific hyperimmune globulin or pooled gamma globulin has been shown to be of added benefit when administered with ganciclovir.[20,21] When Snydman et al. administered CMV immunoglobulin as prophylaxis to CMV-seronegative renal transplant recipients, the incidence of CMV-associated syndromes decreased from 60% to 21%.[22] High-dose oral acyclovir prophylaxis reduced the incidence of CMV disease from 29% to 8% in a randomized trial after renal transplantation.[23] Similar studies must be performed in cardiac allograft recipients before prophylaxis can be recommended.

Herpes Viruses

Herpes viruses other than CMV may also be a source of morbidity owing to reactivation of infection. The treatment of severe herpes simplex or herpes zoster infection consists of high-dose intravenous acyclovir until the lesions have resolved. Prophylaxis with low-dose oral acyclovir is effective in preventing the reactivation of herpes simplex virus infection.[36]

Toxoplasma gondii

Infection with *Toxoplasma gondii* after cardiac transplantation results from either a primary infection, reactivation of a latent infection, or is transmitted via blood products or the donor heart.[24] There are similarities between reactivation of toxoplasmosis and CMV in the immunocompromised host. Reactivation occurs between 4 and 12 weeks after transplantation and is rarely associated with clinically significant disease. In contrast, primary infection has a high frequency of clinical illness. Common manifestations of this infection include encephalitis, myocarditis, and pneumonitis. The pathologic features of myocarditis are only vaguely similar to that of allograft rejection.[25] Inflammatory infiltrates, necrosis, and edema are present but eosinophils are common and should alert the pathologist to search for the cysts, which are diagnostic of infection. Lumbar puncture should be included in the diagnostic work-up for toxoplasmosis because of the high frequency of central nervous system involvement. The treatment of toxoplasmosis is pyrimethamine and sulfadiazine for 6 months.[26] Clindamycin may serve as a substitute for sulfadiazine when the recipient is allergic to sulfonamides.[27]

Human Immunodeficiency Virus

Another infection that can be transmitted through donor organs and blood products is HIV type 1. Blood products and organ donors are routinely screened for HIV antibody. However, a recent infection may not be identified by routine screening. Cohen et al. collected serum samples from 4163 adults who had received more than 36,000 transfusions for cardiac surgery and identified the risk of HIV-1 transmission in screened blood products of approximately 0.003% per unit, suggesting a very low incidence of inadvertent transmission of HIV-1.[28] There have been approximately 20 cases of primary HIV infection transmitted via the blood products or donor organs reported in kidney and liver transplantation.[29] In addition, there have been a similar number of liver and kidney transplants performed in asymptomatic carriers of this virus. Long-term follow-up is not complete; however, the initial impression suggests that the natural history of HIV infection is accelerated in these recipients. An international registry has been established to study the natural history and mode of transmission of HIV infection after transplantation.

Pneumocystis carinii

A common cause of pneumonia in transplant recipients that is not transmitted through blood products or donor organs is *Pneumocystis carinii* (PCP).[30,31] This protozoan produces rapidly progressive interstitial and alveolar pulmonary infiltrates associated with fever and profound hypoxemia. The diagnosis of PCP is made by methenamine silver stain of bronchial secretions. The treatment consists of high-dose trimethoprim/sulfamethoxazole for at least 4 weeks. If treatment is initiated early, the response rate is high. When the pneumonia is resistant, pentamidine has been substituted with good results. Chemoprophylaxis with low-dose trimethoprim/sulfamethoxazole has been shown to prevent the infection.[32] Because trimethoprim/sulfamethoxazole may precipitate leukopenia in patients receiving azathioprine or may be contraindicated in recipients with sulfonamide allergy, inhaled pentamidine prophylaxis may be an alternative.[33]

Legionella pneumophila

Another important cause of pneumonia after cardiac transplantation is *Legionella pneumophila*.[34] This diagnosis is established by direct fluorescent antibody stain of bronchial secretions. The infection usually responds to high-dose intravenous erythromycin, which causes a rise in cyclosporine levels necessitating dose-reduction.

Listeria monocytogenes

Listeria monocytogenes, an enteric bacterium, may cause clinical disease ranging from bacteremia to meningitis.[35] When this organism is identified, high-dose intravenous ampicillin should be administered for 4 to 6 weeks.

Nocardia asteroides

Fungal infections may occur when high-dose prolonged immunosuppression is required. Mucocutaneous candidiasis is an exception to this rule and in general may be prevented with clotrimazole or nystatin oral preparations.[37] *Nocardia asteroides,* a soil-borne aerobic Actinomycetaceae, may be a pathogen in the transplant population and presents as pulmonary, central nervous system, or ocular infection.[38] When evaluation of a solitary pulmonary nodule reveals nocardiosis, a 1-year course of sulfisoxazole is indicated.

Aspergillus

In the severely immunocompromised host, *Aspergillus* infection may be a terminal event. When aspergillosis is invasive, the likelihood of successful treatment is low. Amphotericin B, the drug of choice, is highly toxic to the kidneys and bone marrow, thereby limiting successful treatment. Recently, however, a liposome-encapsulated formulation of amphotericin B, which greatly reduces toxicity, has resulted in successful treatment of invasive aspergillosis.[39,40]

The outcome after transplantation can only be improved when the infectious complications are reduced. The ideal resolution is highly specific immunosuppression. Since such agents have not been developed, minimizing immunosuppression should be considered. Immunosuppressive strategies vary widely among programs but are almost equally divided between those that induce immunosuppression with antilymphocyte antibodies and those that use conventional triple drug immunosuppression for this purpose. At the UTAH Cardiac Transplant Program we have used induction with antilymphocyte antibodies in the hope that long-term high-dose immunosuppression can be avoided. To investigate the role of different types of antilymphocyte antibodies, a prospective trial was conducted comparing a murine anti-CD3 monoclonal antibody (OKT3) immunosuppressive protocol to a polyclonal equine antithymocyte globulin (ATG) protocol.[41] OKT3 had a beneficial effect on rejection while the infection frequency was identical in both groups, with pulmonary infections being the predominant complication. In the OKT3 group, 88% were weaned off corticosteroid maintenance compared to 46% in the ATG group. The infection rate in the patients free of maintenance corticosteroids was approximately $\frac{1}{2}$ that of those continuing to require corticosteroids for maintenance immunosuppression.[42] Oh et al. reported increased infections when OKT3 was used to treat rejection compared to high-dose corticosteroids and antilymphoblast globulin.[43] In contrast, Munda et al. did not observe increased infection after OKT3 treatment for rejection.[44] Singh et al. associated disseminated primary CMV infection to OKT3 rejection therapy.[45] Symptomatic reactivation of herpes simplex was observed in 53% of seropositive recipients who received OKT3 and 31% of those who did not. Hosenpud et al. reported 23 infections in 42 patients undergoing cardiac transplantation (0.5 episodes per patient) using maintenance triple therapy and low-dose corticosteroids for acute rejection.[46] Although it is likely that potent antilymphocyte therapy predisposes recipients to infection, the role of OKT3 specifically in these infections has not been established. A randomized comparison of OKT3 induced immunosuppression to conventional triple therapy-induced immunosuppression in cardiac transplantation is necessary to resolve these issues.[47]

A common clinical problem encountered by transplant physicians is the febrile allograft recipient. An aggressive approach to the diagnosis and treatment of infections is necessary to prevent morbidity and mortality. Fever (temperature >100.5°F), although blunted by corticosteroids, remains the hallmark of infection and warrants an urgent evaluation. Medical history and physical examination should be performed, concentrating on the localizing features of the fever and characteristics that suggest viral versus bacterial infection. Even if no focal findings are identified, a complete blood count with differential, chest x-ray, and cultures of blood, urine, and sputum for routine pathogens as well as CMV are indicated. If neurologic signs are present, computerized axial tomography and lumbar puncture should be performed. When fever and gastrointestinal symptoms are present in a patient at risk for primary CMV, endoscopy with brushing for culture and staining for inclusion bodies may be indicated.

Arterial blood gases should be obtained if the patient complains of dyspnea. Hypoxemia (>10% reduction in baseline arterial Po_2) or a new pulmonary infiltrate necessitate invasive pulmonary diagnosis. Although open-lung biopsy and transtracheal aspiration have been effective diagnostic procedures, bronchoscopy with bronchoalveolar lavage is the most commonly accepted approach to the diagnosis of opportunistic pulmonary infections. Antibiotics should be initiated once the diagnostic procedures have been completed. At the UTAH Cardiac Transplant Program, erythromycin and trimethoprim/sulfamethoxazole are administered if Legionella and Pneumocystis are suspected. It is easy to withdraw therapy if diagnostic studies rule out these infections but valuable time may be lost if therapy is not initiated early. Although ganciclovir is the agent of choice for CMV pneumonia, its toxicities warrant documentation of invasive CMV before initiating its use. A close working relationship among pulmonology, infectious diseases, and the cardiac transplant team is necessary to successfully treat these infections. Infections in an immunocompromised host may be abrupt in onset with rapid progression, and if the experience of the entire team is not recruited, the outcome may be fatal.

Hypertension

Soon after the clinical introduction of cyclosporine, it was recognized that most patients develop systemic hypertension after transplantation (Table 11.4). The hypertension associated with cyclosporine therapy differs clinically from essential hypertension in that there is a loss of the normal circadian variation; that is, blood pressure is equally elevated during the

TABLE 11.4. Characteristics of cyclosporine-induced hypertension.

Mechanisms	Treatment
Sodium retention	Converting enzyme inhibition
Normal plasma renin activity	Calcium channel blockers
Direct vasoconstriction	Beta blockers

night as it is during the day.[48,49] When Thompson et al. compared hemo-dynamic changes after cardiac transplantation in patients receiving "conventional" (azathioprine and prednisone) immunosuppression to those receiving cyclosporine, cardiac output rose equally in both groups, whereas systemic vascular resistance remained elevated only in the cyclosporine group.[50] Cyclosporine-induced hypertension in human subjects is volume-dependent because of sodium retention and is associated with normal plasma renin activity.[51,52] Cyclosporine also directly causes vasoconstriction in isolated vascular smooth muscle.[53] The hypertensive effect of cyclosporine is independent of the nephrotoxicity.

The treatment of cyclosporine-induced hypertension is not standardized. Although diuretics may be effective in theory, hypertension is rarely controlled by diuretics alone. Converting enzyme inhibitors have been used successfully as first-line therapy despite normal or low plasma renin activity; in 60% of recipients they are effective as single agents.[54] Diltiazem is effective and has the additional benefit of increasing cyclosporine levels, which lower cyclosporine requirement and, hence, lower the cost of immunosuppressive therapy.[55] Other calcium channel blockers, such as nicardipine, nifedipine, and verapamil, have been used for hypertension. Unfortunately, large trials have not been performed for any of the regularly used agents in the cardiac transplant population. Therefore, the ideal combination of antihypertensive agents is unknown.

Gastrointestinal Complications

The primary esophageal complication is fungal and/or viral infection primarily with *Candida albicans* or herpes simplex. Esophagitis presents with pain or difficulty in swallowing. An aggressive diagnostic assessment with endoscopy and biopsy is required to establish the diagnosis. Acyclovir is the treatment for herpes simplex infections. Oral nystatin, clotrimazole, or when more serious, intravenous amphotericin, are the therapies for Candida esophagitis.

Gastritis and peptic ulceration are common and may be caused by the combination of corticosteroids, stress, and the aspirin that is frequently administered for the antiplatelet effect. At any sign of upper gastrointestinal pain and/or bleeding, early endoscopy followed by aggressive therapy with H-2 blockers, locally acting agents such as sucralfate, and antacids are required.

The lower gastrointestinal tract may also be affected by ulcerative disease, primarily in association with CMV infection. Perforation of diverticuli may be masked by the effects of corticosteroids and may be unrecognized by all except the astute clinician. Colonic ileus may occur with administration of vincristine and cathartics should be employed to maintain normal bowel movements if this agent is administered.

Hepatitis B, a complication of blood transfusion, may occur after cardiac transplantation. Additionally, azathioprine and cyclophosphamide are hepatotoxic with an additive effect on abnormalities in liver function.[56] Cyclosporine also has dose-dependent hepatotoxicity, which can be avoided by monitoring cyclosporine blood levels. When hepatitis occurs, it must be kept in mind that azathioprine is converted to 6-mercaptopurine by the liver and abnormalities in synthetic function may retard activation of this agent. Prednisone is converted to its active compound prednisolone in the liver and substitution should be considered if there are severe abnormalities of hepatic function. Corticosteroid therapy results in lithogenic bile and cholelithiasis. Pancreatitis has been reported in 8% of autopsied patients after cardiac transplantation.[57] The cause is multifactorial, including infection (particularly CMV), corticosteroids, azathioprine, cyclosporine, thiazide diuretics, cholelithiasis, and low flow states due to extracorporeal circulation or vasopressors.

In our institution, 26 of 173 cardiac transplant recipients (15%) experienced major abdominal complications, including gastrointestinal bleeding (24%), pancreatitis (24%), bowel perforation (18%), cholecystitis (12%), and miscellaneous gastrointestinal problems (21%).[58] Surgery was required in 60% and no deaths were caused by gastrointestinal complications.

Renal Dysfunction

Renal function is abnormal in all patients receiving cyclosporine.[59] This observation was a surprise because nephrotoxicity did not occur in the animal model. Two forms of cyclosporine nephrotoxicity may occur after cardiac transplantation: an acute reversible vasoconstrictive form and a chronic form leading to irreversible interstitial fibrosis of unclear etiology. In the early postoperative period, azotemia and oliguria may develop and spontaneously reverse without alteration of cyclosporine dose.[60] When a cyclosporine loading dose of 18 mg/kg was employed, some recipients required hemodialysis because of the severe nephrotoxicity. Others required conversion of cyclosporine to azathioprine after 6 months to 1 year of cyclosporine therapy because of progressive renal dysfunction. Improved techniques of monitoring serum cyclosporine levels have lead to a greater knowledge of drug interactions, which may intensify the nephrotoxicity. Loading doses of cyclosporine have also decreased from

18 mg/kg to 3 to 8 mg/kg, and some centers avoid giving cyclosporine in the perioperative period. Unquestionably, these changes in dose scheduling have lead to a reduction in cyclosporine nephrotoxicity.

Endocrine/Metabolic Complications

Corticosteroids and cyclosporine induce a wide variety of metabolic effects. Hyperglycemia after cardiac transplantation is common, particularly during administration of high-dose corticosteroids. Diabetic patients will predictably have an increase in insulin dosage or require the addition of insulin when their diabetes was controlled by diet and/or oral hypoglycemic agents at baseline. Patients predisposed to diabetes mellitus may become overtly diabetic. In addition to the effects of corticosteroids, cyclosporine is diabetogenic by both the inhibition of glucose-induced insulin secretion and peripheral resistance to insulin utilization. The addition of cyclosporine to corticosteroids increased the incidence of posttransplant hyperglycemia from 9% to 19% in a comparison of azathioprine- and methylprednisolone-treated renal transplant recipients.[61] Recipients who develop hyperglycemia should be instructed on long-term diabetic care because the diabetic state may become permanent. The use of pulse corticosteroid for the treatment of rejection requires close diabetic surveillance.

Another well known complication of corticosteroid therapy is osteoporosis, characterized by increased bone resorption and impaired bone formation. This side effect can be devastating, resulting in vertebral compression fractures, which dramatically alter rehabilitative potential. In general, postmenopausal women are at highest risk for this complication. Although evidence is lacking, many programs employ vitamin D, calcium, and low-dose estrogen to aid in the prevention of osteoporosis. The success of therapy may depend on the dosage required for corticosteroid maintenance.

Another skeletal complication of corticosteroids is osteonecrosis (aseptic necrosis). This most commonly involves the hip, followed in frequency by the knees and shoulders. In contrast to other causes of osteonecrosis that lead to vascular ischemia (i.e., sickle cell disease), the mechanism by which corticosteroids induce this pathology is unknown. The incidence of osteonecrosis in renal transplant patients has been reported as high as 20%.[62] Patients usually present with pain with weight-bearing or movement of the involved joint. The current diagnostic procedure of choice is magnetic resonance imaging. Initial treatment is symptomatic; ultimately it is joint replacement.

Another musculoskeletal manifestation of chronic corticosteroid usage is growth retardation in children.[63] Despite the severity of this problem, there have been few careful analyses of pituitary hormone secretion in corticosteroid-treated transplant recipients. Growth hormone or soma-tomedin C have not proven valuable in amelioration of this problem. Reduction of corticosteroid dosage should be considered to minimize the growth retardation.

Reproductive function is altered very little after cardiac transplantation.[64,65] Although high-dose corticosteroid therapy results in abnormalities in menstrual and sexual function, fertility may not be affected. The risks of pregnancy include intolerance to the hemodynamic requirements of pregnancy, the teratogenic effects of immunosuppressive therapy, and risk of rejection owing to the immunologic alterations of pregnancy. The ethical issue regarding pregnancy in a woman with reduced life expectancy must be considered individually by the transplant physician and the recipient. The effect of immunosuppression on fertility is unknown in men. If spermatogenesis is grossly abnormal, the product of conception will not be viable and spontaneous abortion will occur. There are no reports addressing the effect of immunosuppression on male reproductive function in human subjects.

It is likely that the cardiac allograft will successfully adapt to the changes in preload and afterload of pregnancy, labor, and delivery. Corticosteroids and azathioprine have no known teratogenic effects. Methotrexate and cyclophosphamide are known to have teratogenic effects and should not be administered during pregnancy. The teratogenicity of cyclosporine is unknown. There are case reports of successful pregnancies in renal transplant recipients receiving cyclosporine. However, anencephaly, an increased incidence of spontaneous miscarriages, and the complete absence of the corpus callosum have been described.[64]

There is some evidence to suggest that certain placental proteins may directly affect suppressor lymphocyte function and thereby theoretically prevent immunologic responses to fetal antigens during pregnancy.[66] Although a change in the frequency of rejection has not been reported in pregnant renal transplant recipients, it is unclear how these immunologic alterations may affect the recipient's response to the allograft. Lowenstein et al. reported a successful pregnancy in a cardiac transplant recipient who did not show an increased incidence of rejection, although cyclosporine levels fluctuated widely.[67] The child was normal. It is recommended that cardiac transplant recipients do not become pregnant and oral contraception and/or tubal ligation be seriously considered.

Lipid metabolism is also altered by immunosuppressive therapy. Corticosteroids induce an elevation in serum cholesterol.[68] Cyclosporine impairs low density lipoprotein hepatic clearance, which results in hypercholesterolemia.[69]

Although the role of hyperlipidemia in the development of cardiac allograft vasculopathy is debated, approximately 30% of patients undergoing cardiac transplantation were victims of coronary artery disease with refractory left ventricular dysfunction.[4] Since atherosclerosis is a systemic disease, control of cholesterol may retard the progression of atherosclerosis that is invariably present in the aorta and peripheral and cerebral vasculatures. Patients in whom corticosteroids are either minimized or totally discontinued show significantly lower serum cholesterol levels than patients requiring high-dose corticosteroids.[70] In our experience, patients free of maintenance corticosteroids had a 26% lower fasting serum cholesterol level during the first 18 months after cardiac transplantation, with a mean serum cholesterol of 200 mg% in patients not requiring corticosteroid maintenance compared to 270 mg% in corticosteroid-dependent recipients.[71]

Treatment of hypercholesterolemia should include intensive weight loss, rigorous dietary restriction, and hypolipidemic agents. In our program, first-line therapy consists of gemfibrozil, 600 to 1200 mg/day. Bile acid binding agents, although effective, are less well tolerated and may alter cyclosporine absorption. Lovastatin is effective in the treatment of hypercholesterolemia by the inhibition of cholesterol synthesis as a 3-hydroxy-3-methyglutaryl-coenzyme A (HMG-CoA) reductase inhibitor. However, when this agent is combined with cyclosporine, lovastatin levels increase and the toxicity is accentuated. This has resulted in renal injury due to rhabdomyolysis.[72] In addition, this effect is potentiated by concomitant gemfibrozil therapy. Lovastatin can be used in selected patients with severe, poorly controlled hypercholesterolemia only when low doses are initiated (10–20 mg/day), serum creatine kinase is monitored serially, and the agent is discontinued at the first sign of liver dysfunction and/or elevation in the muscle enzymes.[73]

Neurologic Complications

Seizures have been observed in as many as 15% of recipients and are multifactorial in origin.[74] Patients with severe left ventricular dysfunction before transplant and subtherapeutic anticoagulation may experience embolic cerebral vascular events that heal by scar formation, serving as a potential focus for seizures. Wide fluctuations in arterial pressure, arrhythmias, and metabolic disturbances may also occur after cardiac transplantation. In addition, cyclosporine lowers seizure threshold. When a patient has a seizure after cardiac transplantation, a detailed evaluation including tomographic imaging and lumbar puncture should be performed to rule out undisclosed focal neurologic lesions and infection. Metabolic abnormalities such as hypomagnesemia should be corrected and anticonvulsant therapy should be instituted.

Diphenylhydantoin remains the cornerstone of maintenance anticonvulsive therapy. However, because this agent induces the P-450 hepatic enzyme system, cyclosporine metabolism is accelerated, requiring an increase in dose. This may also be true for azathioprine and prednisone. The appropriate duration of anticonvulsant therapy is unknown. Our policy has been to maintain anticonvulsant therapy indefinitely; however, this is controversial.

Malignancy

Immunosuppressive therapy promotes the development of malignancies after cardiac transplantation. Transplant recipients have a 6% risk of developing a malignant tumor, which represents an age-controlled frequency 100 times greater than the general population.[75] Malignant tumors have also been found in patients who received immunosuppression over prolonged periods for indications other than transplantation; hence, the immune system modification or the direct carcinogenicity of the agents and not the transplanted organ predisposes to malignancy. Lymphoma, skin cancer, and Kaposi's sarcoma have been reported at higher frequency in this population. Because of the high incidence of skin cancers, transplant patients should be followed carefully by dermatologists and protection from solar injury should be routine.

Cyclosporine in combination with rabbit antithymocyte globulin predisposed cardiac transplant recipients to lymphoma during the initial clinical trials.[76] A reduction in cyclosporine dosage and attenuation of rabbit antithymocyte globulin has decreased the incidence to 0.4%.[77]

Lymphomas are distributed in an atypical pattern after transplantation. Primary cerebral and gastrointestinal lymphomas are common presentations. Early lymphomatous lesions have been shown to be polyclonal and associated with Epstein-Barr virus infection.[78] It has been postulated that these lymphomas arise from polyclonal B-cell proliferation in response to virus infection. Patients who present with an infectious mononucleosis-like syndrome with polyclonal, morphologically benign B-cell proliferation without cytogenetic abnormalities respond to acyclovir.[79] In contrast, solid tumors that are monoclonal and morphologically malignant are not responsive to acyclovir. When a transplant patient has a fever of undetermined etiology or constitutional symptoms that cannot be explained and the Epstein-Barr virus titer is elevated, lymphoma should be considered. The evaluation consists of careful assessment of the gastrointestinal tract and the central nervous system with tissue diagnosis of suspicious lesions for histology and lymphocyte phenotype. If the lymphoma consists of monoclonal B cells, minimizing immunosuppression, chemotherapy, and radiation should be considered. If it is polyclonal, a trial of high-dose intravenous acyclovir is warranted.

Cardiac Allograft Vasculopathy

Each of the medical complications discussed thus far in this chapter is associated with immunosuppressive therapy. Cardiac allograft vasculopathy (CAV) is a complication that is not directly related to immunosuppression and serves as the major cause of morbidity and mortality after the first year after cardiac transplantation. This form of coronary artery

TABLE 11.5. Cardiac allograft vasculopathy:
Predisposing factors

Immune factors	Atherogenic factors
Cytotoxic B-cell antibodies	Donor age
Lymphocytotoxic HLA–antibodies	Hyperlipidemia
CMV infection	
Rejection frequency?	

disease differs from coronary atherosclerosis in nontransplant patients in that the lesions begin in the microvasculature and involve proximal vessels only when far advanced. Microscopically, concentric intimal proliferation leads to progressive occlusion of the lumen.[80] In some lesions, lipid-laden macrophages may be seen.

Because the heart is denervated, patients with CAV will not experience anginal symptoms. The presenting manifestations are unexplained left ventricular dysfunction owing to diffuse ischemia or arrhythmia. The diagnostic standard for the detection of CAV remains coronary arteriography; however, interpretation of coronary angiograms in the early phase is difficult because there may be only a diffuse narrowing of the coronary tree or an abrupt cut-off of a tertiary branch of a coronary artery. As a result, many institutions perform baseline coronary angiography to measure luminal diameter for comparison to serial studies. Because this lesion occurs initially in microscopic vessels, occasionally endomyocardial biopsy may provide a clue to the diagnosis.[81] Other noninvasive tests, including treadmill exercise performance, thallium perfusion, and Holter monitoring, do not lend sufficient sensitivity and specificity to be considered effective screening tests. The hypotensive response to exercise has been suggested as a valuable clue to CAV.[82]

Uretsky et al. reported the prevalence of CAV as 18% at 1 year and 44% at 3 years.[83] Similarly, Gao et al. noted a 14% incidence in the first year and 50% by 5 years in cyclosporine-treated patients.[84] In our experience, the incidence of CAV was 17% at one year and 25% at 2 years.[85] However, only one-third of these angiograms showed severe (>50% luminal narrowing) disease in any vessel.

The immunopathogenesis of CAV is poorly understood. It is widely accepted that the lesion represents immune-mediated injury with increased vascular permeability leading to lipid deposition if an atherogenic milieu is present (Table 11.5). The first reported predisposing risk factors to CAV included donor age, with older donors (21 vs. 24 years of age) showing a higher incidence of disease and elevated plasma triglycerides.[80] The presence of cytotoxic B-cell antibodies,[86] hypercholesterolemia,[86] lymphocytotoxic human leukocyte antigen (HLA) antibodies,[87] and CMV infection[88] have all been correlated to the development of allograft vasculopathy. Surprisingly, rejection has not consistently correlated with

CAV, possibly because the pathogenesis of the myocyte directed, cell-mediated rejection typically diagnosed by biopsy differs from the immune-mediated vascular injury that leads to CAV. Immunosuppressive protocols have been compared and the addition of cyclosporine does not affect the incidence of CAV. In addition, we have not found a difference in polyclonal (ATG) versus monoclonal (OKT3) T-cell agents as a predisposing factor for CAV.[85] However, withdrawal of corticosteroids may safely be attempted because there is no difference in incidence of CAV in those patients withdrawn from maintenance corticosteroids compared to those requiring corticosteroids.

It had been hoped that CAV could be prevented with the addition of antiplatelet agents. Griepp et al. published an enthusiastic report that warfarin and dipyridamole, in addition to weight reduction and maintenance of the low cholesterol, low fat diet, retarded the development of "coronary atherosclerosis".[89] Unfortunately, these results have not been confirmed in large scale follow-up studies. Yet, many centers continue to administer antiplatelet agents routinely.

When there are discrete lesions of proximal coronary arteries (distinctly unusual), angioplasty has seen limited success.[90] Unfortunately, the only proven therapy for CAV is retransplantation. In the Stanford series, the 1-year survival after retransplantation was markedly decreased compared to first operations at 55%.[91]

Conclusion

The medical complications that follow cardiac transplantation encompass a wide spectrum of organ systems and require the input of multiple specialists. Most can be minimized with careful monitoring of immunosuppressive therapy and are generally preventable. The primary cardiac transplant physician and personnel should be familiar with these complications and institute early aggressive diagnostic procedures and therapy where appropriate.

Cardiac allograft vasculopathy for which the diagnostic standards are inadequate and therapy is essentially nonexistent remains the limiting factor to long-term survival. Future research directed toward improving outcome in cardiac transplantation should be focused toward a better understanding of the immunopathogenesis and prevention of cardiac allograft vasculopathy.

References

1. O'Connell JB, Renlund DG, Bristow MR. Cardiac transplantation: emerging role of the internist/cardiologist. *J Intern Med.* 1989;225:147–156.
2. Hosenpud JD, Morton MJ. Hemodynamic assessment and physiology of the

transplanted heart. In: Hosenpud JD, Cobanoglu A, Norman D, Starr A, eds. *Cardiac Transplantation: A Manual for Health Care Professionals and Trainees*. New York, NY: Springer-Verlag. In press.

3. O'Connell JB, Renlund DG, Lee HR, et al. Newer techniques of immunosuppression in cardiac transplantation. *Cardiac Surgery: State of the Art Reviews* 1988;2:607–615.

4. Fragomeni LS, Kaye, MP. The Registry of the International Society for Heart Transplantation: fifth official report—1988. *J Heart Transplant*. 1988;7:249–253.

5. Mason JW, Stinson EB, Hunt SA, et al. Infections after cardiac transplantation: relation to rejection therapy. *Ann Intern Med*. 1976;85:69–72.

6. Hofflin JA, Potasman I, Baldwin JC, et al. Infectious complications in heart transplant recipients receiving cyclosporine and corticosteroids. *Ann Intern Med*. 1987;106:209–216.

7. Dresdale AR, Drusin RE, Lamb J, et al. Reduced infection in cardiac transplant recipients. *Circulation*. 1985;72(suppl II):237–240.

8. Report of the Working Group of Transplant Cardiologists, Chicago, Ill 1989. Unpublished.

9. Trento A, Dummer GS, Hardesty RL. Mediastinitis following heart transplantation: incidence, treatment, and results. *Heart Transplant*. 1984;3:336–340.

10. Miller R, Ruder J, Karwande SV, et al. Treatment of mediastinitis after heart transplantation. *J Heart Transplant*. 1986;5:477–479.

11. Gottesdiener KM. Transplanted infections: donor-to-host transmission with the allograft. *Ann Intern Med*. 1989;110:1001–1016.

12. Guttendorf J, Bohachick P, Dummer JS, et al. The impact of protective isolation on the incidence of early infection in adult heart transplant patients. *Circulation*. 1988;78(suppl II):II-3. Abstract.

13. Dummer JS, White LT, Ho M, et al. Morbidity of cytomegalovirus infection in recipients of heart or heart-lung transplants who received cyclosporine. *J Infect Dis*. 1985;152:1182–1191.

14. Collier AC, Chandler SH, Handsfield HH, et al. Identification of multiple strains of cytomegalovirus in homosexual men. *J Infect Dis*. 1989;159:123–126.

15. Smith CB. Cytomegalovirus pneumonia state of the art. *Chest*. 1989;95(suppl):182S–187S.

16. Bloom JN, Palestine AG. The diagnosis of cytomegalovirus retinitis. *Ann Intern Med*. 1988;109:963–969.

17. Gonwa TA, Capehart JE, Pilcher JW, et al. Cytomegalovirus myocarditis as a cause of cardiac dysfunction in a heart transplant recipient. *Transplantation*. 1989;47:197–199.

18. Watson FS, O'Connell JB, Amber IJ, et al. Treatment of cytomegalovirus pneumonia in heart transplant recipients with 9(1,3-dihydroxy-2-proproxy-methyl)-guanine (DHPG). *J Heart Transplant*. 1988;7:102–105.

19. Keay S, Petersen E, Icenogle T, et al. Ganciclovir treatment of serious cytomegalovirus infection in heart and heart-lung transplant recipients. *Rev Infect Dis*. 1988;10(suppl 3):S563–S572.

20. Reed EC, Bowden RA, Dandliker PS, et al. Treatment of cytomegalovirus pneumonia with ganciclovir and intravenous cytomegalovirus immunoglobu-

lin in patients with bone marrow transplants. *Ann Intern Med.* 1988;109:783–788.

21. Emanuel D, Cunningham I, Jules-Elysee K, et al. Cytomegalovirus pneumonia after bone marrow transplantation successfully treated with the combination of ganciclovir and high-dose intravenous immune globulin. *Ann Intern Med.* 1988;109:777–782.

22. Snydman DR, Werner BG, Heinze-Lacey B, et al. Use of cytomegalovirus immune globulin to prevent cytomegalovirus disease in renal-transplant recipients. *N Engl J Med.* 1987;317:1049–1054.

23. Balfour HH, Chace BA, Stapleton JT, et al. A randomized, placebo-controlled trial of oral acyclovir for the prevention of cytomegalovirus disease in recipients of renal allografts. *N Engl J Med.* 1989;320:1381–1387.

24. Luft BJ, Naot Y, Araujo F, et al. Primary and reactivated toxoplasma infection in patients with cardiac transplant. *Ann Intern Med.* 1983;99:27–31.

25. Luft BJ, Billingham M, Remington JS. Endomyocardial biopsy in the diagnosis of toxoplasmic myocarditis. *Transplant Proc.* 1986;18:1871–1873.

26. Leport C, Raffi F, Matheron S, et al. Treatment of central nervous system toxoplasmosis with pyrimethamine/sulfadiazine combination in 35 patients with the acquired immunodeficiency syndrome. *Am J Med.* 1988;84:94–100.

27. Dannemann BR, Israelski DM, Remington JS. Treatment of toxoplasmic encephalitis with intravenous clindamycin. *Arch Intern Med.* 1988;148:2477–2482.

28. Cohen ND, Munoz A, Reitz BA, et al. Transmission of retroviruses by transfusion of screened blood in patients undergoing cardiac surgery. *N Engl J Med.* 1989;320:1172–1176.

29. Rubin RH, Tolkoff-Rubin NE. The problem of human immunodeficiency virus (HIV) infection and transplantation. *Transplant Int.* 1988;1:36–42.

30. Peters SG, Prakash UBS. Pneumocystis carinii pneumonia. *Am J Med.* 1987;82:73–78.

31. Franson RT, Kauffman HM Jr, Adams MB, et al. Cyclosporine therapy and refractory Pneumocystis carinii pneumonia. *Arch Surg.* 1987;122:1034–1035.

32. Higgins RM, Bloom SL, Hopkin JM, et al. The risks and benefits of low-dose cotrimoxazole prophylaxis for Pneumocystis pneumonia in renal transplantation. *Transplantation.* 1989;47:558–560.

33. Golden JA, Chernoff D, Hollander H, et al. Prevention of Pneumocystis carinii pneumonia by inhaled pentamidine. *Lancet.* 1989;l:654–657.

34. Favor A, Frazier OH, Cooley DA, et al. Legionella infections in cyclosporine-immunosuppressed cardiac transplants. *Tex Heart Inst J.* 1985;12:153–156.

35. Marget W, Seeliger HPR. Listeria monocytogenes infections-therapeutic possibilities and problems. *Infection.* 1988;16(suppl 2):S175–S177.

36. Seale L, Jones CJ, Kathpalia S, et al. Prevention of herpesvirus infections in renal allograft recipients by low-dose oral acyclovir. *JAMA.* 1985;254:3435–3438.

37. Gombert ME, duBouchet L, Aulicino TM, et al. A comparative trial of clotrimazole troches and oral nystatin suspension in recipients of renal transplants. *JAMA.* 1987;258:2553–2555.

38. Wilson JP, Turner HR, Kirchner KA, et al. Nocardia infections in renal transplant recipients. *Medicine.* 1989;68:38–53.

39. Wiebe VJ, DeGregorio MW. Liposome-encapsulated amphotericin B: a promising new treatment for disseminated fungal infections. *Rev Infect Dis.* 1988;10:1097–1101.
40. Radovancevic B, Frazier OH, Gentry LO, et al. Successful treatment of invasive aspergillosis in a heart transplant patient. *Tex Heart Inst J.* 1985;12:233–237.
41. Renlund DG, O'Connell JB, Gilbert EM, et al. A prospective comparison of murine monoclonal CD-3 (OKT3) antibody-based and equine antithymocyte globulin-based rejection prophylaxis in cardiac transplantation. *Transplantation.* 1989;47:599–605.
42. Renlund DG, O'Connell JB, Gilbert EM, et al. Feasibility of discontinuation of corticosteroid maintenance therapy in heart transplantation. *J Heart Transplant.* 1987;6:71–78.
43. Oh CH, Stratta RB, Fox BC, et al. Increased infections associated with the use of OKT3 for treatment of steroid- resistant rejection in renal transplantation. *Transplantation.* 1988;45:68–73.
44. Munda R, Hutchins M, First MR, et al. Infection in OKT3-treated patients receiving additional antirejection therapy. *Transplant Proc.* 1989;21:1763–1765.
45. Singh N, Dummer JS, Kusne S, et al. Infections with cytomegalovirus and other herpesviruses in 121 liver transplant recipients: transmission by donated organ and the effect of OKT3 antibodies. *J Infect Dis.* 1988;158:124–131.
46. Hosenpud JD, Norman DJ, Pantley GA, et al. Low morbidity and mortality from infection following cardiac transplantation using maintenance triple therapy and low-dose corticosteroids for acute rejection. *Clin Transplant.* 1988;2:201–206.
47. Renlund DG, O'Connell JB, Bristow MR. Early rejection prophylaxis in heart transplantation: Is cytolytic therapy necessary? *J Heart Transplant.* 1989;8:191–193.
48. Wenting GJ, Van den Meiracker AH, Ritsema van Eck HJ, et al. Lack of circadian variation of blood pressure after heart transplantation. *J Hypertension.* 1986;4(suppl 6):S78–S80.
49. Reeves RA, Shapiro AP, Thompson ME, et al. Loss of nocturnal decline in blood pressure after cardiac transplantation. *Circulation.* 1986;73:401–408.
50. Thompson ME, Shapiro AP, Johnsen AM, et al. The contrasting effects of cyclosporin-A and azathioprine on arterial blood pressure and renal function following cardiac transplantation. *Int J Cardiol.* 1986;11:219–229.
51. Curtis JJ, Luke RG, Jones P, et al. Hypertension in cyclosporine-treated renal transplant recipients is sodium dependent. *Am J Med.* 1988;85:134–138.
52. Bantle JP, Boudreau RJ, Ferris TF. Suppression of plasma renin activity by cyclosporine. *Am J Med.* 1987;83:59–64.
53. Bennett WM, Porter GA. Cyclosporine-associated hypertension. *Am J Med.* 1988;85:131–133.
54. Jessup M, Cavarocchi N, Narins B, et al. Antihypertensive therapy in patients after cardiac transplantation: a step-care approach. *Transplant Proc.* 1988;20(suppl 1):801–802.
55. Ratkovec RM, Renlund DG, Bristow MR, et al. Diltiazem treatment of cyclosporine-induced hypertension after cardiac transplantation. *Cardiovasc Drugs Ther.* 1989;3:622. Abstract.

56. Shaunak S, Munro JM, Weinbren K, et al. Cyclophosphamide-induced liver necrosis: a possible interaction with azathioprine. *Q J Med* 1988;67:309–317.
57. Aziz S, Bergdahl L, Baldwin JC, et al. Pancreatitis after cardiac and cardiopulmonary transplantation. *Surgery*. 1985;97:653–661.
58. Merrell SW, Ames SA, Nelson EW, et al. Major abdominal complications following cardiac transplantation. *Arch Surg*. 1989;124:889–894.
59. Meyers BD, Ross J, Newton L, et al. Cyclosporine-associated chronic nephropathy. *N Engl J Med*. 1984;311:699–705.
60. Greenberg A, Egel JW, Thompson ME, et al. Early and late forms of cyclosporine nephrotoxicity: studies in cardiac transplant recipients. *Am J Kidney Dis*. 1987;9:12–22.
61. Roth D, Milgrom M, Esquenazi V, et al. Posttransplant hyperglycemia. *Transplantation*. 1989;47:278–281.
62. Ibels LS, Alfrey AC, Huffer WE, Weil R. Aseptic necrosis of bone after renal transplantation: experience in 194 transplant recipients and review of the literature. *Medicine*. 1978;57:25–45.
63. Hyams JS, Carey DE. Corticosteroids and growth. *J Pediatr*. 1988;113:249–254.
64. Kossoy LR, Herbert CM, Wentz AC. Management of heart transplant recipients: guidelines for the obstetrician-gynecologist. *Am J Obstet Gynecol*. 1988;159:490–499.
65. Yeast JD. Immunosuppressives in pregnant transplant patients—what risks? *Contemp OB/GYN*. 1987;30:117–124.
66. Bolton AE, Pockley AG, Clough KU, et al. Identification of placental protein 14 as an immunosuppressive factor in human reproduction. *Lancet*. 1987;1:593–595.
67. Lowenstein BR, Vain NW, Perrone SV, et al. Successful pregnancy and vaginal delivery after heart transplantation. *Am J Obstet Gynecol*. 1988;158:589–590.
68. Zimmerman J, Fainaru M, Eisenberg S. The effects of prednisone therapy on plasma lipoproteins and apolipoproteins: a prospective study. *Metabolism*. 1984;33:521–526.
69. Stamler JS, Vaughan DE, Rudd MA, et al. Frequency of hypercholesterolemia after cardiac transplantation. *Am J Cardiol*. 1988;62:1268–1272.
70. Becker DM, Chamberlain B, Swank R, et al. Relationship between corticosteroid exposure and plasma lipid levels in heart transplant recipients. *Am J Med*. 1988;85:632–638.
71. Renlund DG, Bristow MR, Crandall BG, et al. Hypercholesterolemia after heart transplantation: amelioration by corticosteroid-free maintenance immunosuppression. *J Heart Transplant*. 1989;8:214–220.
72. Corpier CL, Jones PH, Suki WN, et al. Rhabdomyolysis and renal injury with lovastatin use. *JAMA*. 1988;260:239–241.
73. Miller LW, Noedel N, Pennington DG. Treatment of hypercholesterolemia in cardiac transplant recipients with lovastatin. Presented to the 8th Annual Meeting of the American Society of Transplant Physicians Chicago, Ill; 1989. Abstract.
74. Grigg MM, Costanzo-Nordin MR, Celesia GG, et al. The etiology of seizures after cardiac transplantation. *Transplant Proc*. 1988;20(suppl 3):937–944.

75. Penn I. Malignancies associated with immunosuppressive or cytotoxic therapy. *Surgery*. 1978;83:492–502.
76. Anderson JL, Fowles RE, Bieber CP, et al. Idiopathic cardiomyopathy, age, and suppressor-cell dysfunction as risk determinants of lymphoma after cardiac transplantation. *Lancet*. 1978;2:1174–1177.
77. Penn I. Cancers following cyclosporine therapy. *Transplantation*. 1987;43:32–35.
78. Cleary ML, Sklar J. Lymphoproliferative disorders in cardiac transplant recipients are multiclonal lymphomas. *Lancet*. 1984;2:491–493.
79. Hanto DW, Gajl-Peczalska KJ, Balfour HH, et al. Acyclovir therapy of Epstein-Barr virus-induced posttransplant lymphoproliferative diseases. *Transplant Proc*. 1985;17:89–92.
80. Billingham ME. Cardiac transplant atherosclerosis. *Transplant Proc*. 1987;19(suppl 5):19–25.
81. Palmer DC, Tsai CC, Roodman ST, et al. Heart graft arteriosclerosis—an ominous finding on endomyocardial biopsy. *Transplantation*. 1985;39:385–388.
82. Valantine HA, Mullin AV, Hunt SA, et al. Detection of accelerated graft atherosclerosis: importance of hemodynamic response to exercise. *Circulation*. 1988;78(suppl II):II-252. Abstract.
83. Uretsky BF, Murali S, Reddy PS, et al. Development of coronary artery disease in cardiac transplant patients receiving immunosuppressive therapy with cyclosporine and prednisone. *Circulation*. 1987;76:827–834.
84. Gao SZ, Schroeder J, Alderman E, et al. Incidence of accelerated coronary artery disease in heart transplant survivors: comparison of cyclosporin and azathioprine regimen. *Circulation*. 1988;78(suppl II):II-280. Abstract.
85. Ratkovec RM, Wray RB, Renlund DG, et al. Corticosteroid-free maintenance immunosuppression in allograft coronary artery disease following cardiac transplantation. *J Thorac Cardiovasc Surg*. 1990;100:6–12.
86. Hess ML, Hastillo A, Mohanakumar T, et al. Accelerated atherosclerosis in cardiac transplantation: role of cytotoxic B- cell antibodies and hyperlipidemia. *Circulation*. 1983;68(suppl II):II-94–II-101.
87. Petrossian GA, Hernadi S, Nichols AB, et al. Increased mortality and coronary artery disease in cardiac transplant recipients with lymphocytotoxic anti-HLA antibodies. *Circulation*. 1988;78(suppl II):II-86. Abstract.
88. Grattan MT, Moreno-Cabral CE, Starnes VA, et al. Cytomegalovirus infection is associated with cardiac allograft rejection and atherosclerosis. *JAMA*. 1989;261:3561–3566.
89. Griepp RB, Stinson EB, Bieber CP, et al. Control of graft arteriosclerosis in human heart transplant recipients. *Surgery*. 1977;81:262–269.
90. Vetrovec GW, Cowley MJ, Newton CM, et al. Applications of percutaneous transluminal coronary angioplasty in cardiac transplantation. *Circulation*. 1988;78(suppl III):III-83–III-86.
91. Gao SZ, Schroeder JS, Hunt S, et al. Retransplantation for severe accelerated coronary artery disease in heart transplant recipients. *Am J Cardiol*. 1988;62:876–881.

12
Psychiatric Considerations in the Cardiac Transplant Recipient

ROBERT A. MARICLE

Psychiatric considerations in cardiac transplantation arise from a group of interrelated issues and observations. Throughout the course of transplantation, patients encounter a series of stresses that entail emotional, cognitive, and behavioral adaptation.[1-4] When this process breaks down, the patient's well-being and compliance with medical care are jeopardized. The exclusion of some individuals who seek transplantation, based on psychiatric[2,5,6] or psychosocial[7-9] evidence, attempts to circumvent this problem, despite numerous practical and ethical dilemmas that ensue.[10-13] However, this is often insufficient because many reports of psychopathology or noncompliance come from already "screened" groups.[1,6,14] Thus, comprehensive management of recipients must necessarily include plans to supervise recipient adjustment as well as to recognize and treat a range of psychiatric contingencies. This chapter will briefly review some of these issues, discuss elements of a psychiatric evaluation for transplant candidates, highlight the more serious psychiatric conditions the clinician may confront, and consider cardiac implications of psychotropic drugs.

Stages of Transplantation

Many observers have identified adaptive psychological stages in an individual's progression from transplant applicant to long-term survivor.[1,2,4,15,16] These are often depicted using concepts such as stress and coping, adjustment, adaptation, or bereavement: ubiquitous psychological processes that impinge on each patient regardless of his physical or psychological health. Various generalizations keyed to these stages come from an array of clinicians experienced with transplant patients, but are infrequently validated methodically. Still, the stages do organize typical stressors, dilemmas, and responses in a logical chronology, and a brief illustration of a few of the salient elements follows.

Initial Illness

A series of stresses and responses is initiated as the underlying heart disease develops. Distressing symptoms, disability, and the threat of death demand both the individual's attention and some adaptive reaction. This is similar to other serious illnesses, and landmarks in the psychosocial journey are well described: shock, denial, disbelief, anger, bargaining and magical thinking, depression, and resolution or acceptance.[17]

Recommendation of Transplantation

Obviously, the site in this process at which one considers transplantation may predict the immediate reaction or may simply reiterate the basic sequence.[1,2,4,16] For some, this is complicated further by role changes and financial strains in the family.[3,4] Still, when the topic is seriously raised, many patients initially reject it as too extreme, too frightening, too shocking. But with time to gather more information, most patients reconsider, particularly as physical symptoms progressively worsen. For many patients the decision to go forward becomes a simple one. The choice is between continuing disability, suffering, and imminent death or the chance for an improved quality of life and extended survival; this is succinctly summarized as: "I have no choice."

Evaluation for Transplantation

With the transplant evaluation, ambivalence about the procedure and determination to be selected sometimes collide.[1-4] Of course, candidates are very much aware (perhaps out of proportion) that a selection process is occurring, one in which their lives hang in the balance. Understandably, anxiety is viewed as the predominant emotional state during this stage.[1-3,16]

Waiting

Once selected, the candidate is temporarily relieved and begins the wait for a donor. However, this period may rapidly become "interminable" and is often described as the most difficult stage in the transplant process.[1-3] Confidence and hope are replaced by renewed anxiety, recurring worries that a heart will not be found, worsening symptoms, demoralization, and financial and interpersonal strains for both the patient and his family.[1,3,4,18] Some patients find that help from support groups, counseling, or psychotherapy during this time is useful. Still, doubt and insecurity reign,[4,16] and regularly scheduled visits with the medical staff may bring the only real comfort and reassurance.[19]

Perioperative Period

An organ becomes available and within hours the patient is contacted, prepared for surgery, and anesthetized. This has been well rehearsed by the patient, occurs quickly, and is remembered as relatively easy. Usually, so is the immediate postoperative period, characterized as it is by a "honeymoon" of symptomatic relief, excitement, rejuvenation, and euphoria.[1-4,16,18] However, the looming possibility of rejection eventually begins to produce demoralization in some patients, and psychological regression in others.[2,3,18] Medical complications, boredom, and social isolation may then lead to dependency problems and depression.[1,16,18]

Leaving the Hospital

As the time arrives to prepare to leave the hospital, anxiety reappears,[1,18] perhaps in part due to the amount of psychological regression and dependency inherent in transplant hospitalization. Patients have had constant surveillance and attention by a host of physicians and nurses, have often been kept at the limits of their ability to cope by around-the-clock examinations and treatments, and in the process may have repeatedly concluded there is a substantial risk of one catastrophic event or another. Thus, some perceive the transition to out-patient status as precipitous, risky, and worrisome.

Once outside the hospital, this anxiety and insecurity may be manifested by frequent telephone calls, hypochondriacal behavior, or anger. For a brief time this type of behavior can be managed with reassurance and patience but many patients must eventually be gently confronted with limit-setting. They can be told which phone calls and which complaints are appropriate for urgent attention and which can wait until the next clinic appointment. But it is important to present this matter-of-factly as an educational task and not as a rebuke; one must avoid the judgmental and rejecting response that this kind of behavior elicits.

At many points after the surgery patients express gratitude and altruism by presenting gifts to the transplant staff, by offering time to help the program in any way they can, by giving testimonials to the media, by working with donor procurement organizations, and even by donating supplies to be used by future transplant patients. These are understandable, natural, and healthy responses—as long as they are within limits. However, some patients seem to use this behavior to remain unduly attached to the transplant team, perhaps to avoid re-engaging in the uncertainties and frustrations of everyday life, and to maintain a hypertrophied identity as a heart transplant patient. They may need to be encouraged to disengage gradually, return to work, and focus on their lives away from the transplant program and the institution.

Follow-up

Outcome for most recipients is good in terms of survival, long-term physical and psychological function, quality of life, and return to work.[5,20–24] But, adaptive demands do not end with hospital discharge. It is not easy for recipients to resume their former roles in the family and their community.[1–3,16] Returning to work is often fraught with major problems outside the patient's control.[4,23] Spouses or partners are prone to develop delayed emotional problems, and ensuing marital problems can arise.[1,4] Troublesome drug side effects, organic impairments, and problems with concentration, emotional lability, and irritability may emerge.[18] Patients with personality disorders or unresolved coping problems may signal that these will be chronic. Worse, noncompliance with medications or medical appointments may develop.

Psychopathology among Transplant Candidates

In addition to the many articles that describe psychosocial problems or mention psychiatric disorders in transplant patients, several reports have delineated findings from initial psychiatric evaluations. Problems with the diagnostic reliability of these conditions as well as their ultimate validation in terms of posttransplant morbidity, natural history, and response to treatment are just beginning to be worked out. But, the number of reports that document significantly jeopardized outcome as a result of problems with adaptation or psychopathology, usually with noncompliance as the cause, is growing.

For instance, in evaluating 69 candidates, Kuhn et al.[25] found 64% had *Diagnostic and Statistical Manual of Mental Disorders, Third Edition* (DSM-III) diagnoses. Although these did not predict postoperative outcome among the 27 who went on to receive grafts, patients with personality disorder diagnoses, substance abuse, and organic brain syndromes required inordinate attention preoperatively and tended to continue to have problems postoperatively. Antisocial personality disorder appeared to be the only categorical exclusion to transplantation. Mai[26] reported on subsets of the 86 candidates (of whom 33 eventually became recipients) in which 39% of 66 received a psychiatric diagnosis, most commonly anxiety. Although data on the prevalence of personality disorder and substance abuse were not presented, the policy of the Mai team was that the co-existence of these two diagnoses represented an "absolute contraindication to surgery". Freeman et al.[6] found 26 patients with Axis I diagnoses (diagnoses other than personality disorder) and five with Axis II (personality disorder) diagnoses among 70 patients undergoing transplantation, and concluded that a preoperative Axis I diagnosis was associated with postoperative dissatisfaction by the recipient about outcome.

Among 70 potential candidates evaluated by Frierson and Lippmann,[14] 13 were denied the procedure on psychiatric grounds, implying significant psychopathology. These conditions were characterized by the following diagnoses: antisocial personality disorder, substance abuse, and intellectual impairments. Another 17 patients had DSM-III diagnoses but went on to be among 43 of the 70 who received hearts. The authors suggest that those with psychiatric disorders had disproportionate problems with clinical management, psychiatric decompensation, and medical problems. In contrast, the impression of Kay and Bienenfeld,[27] based on the 50 cases they evaluated, was that DSM-III diagnoses do not correlate with outcome. They recommend that psychiatric evaluations be supplemented with measures of cooperation, social support, attitudes, and coping apart from formal psychiatric diagnoses. They argue further that disqualifiers for surgery should be established by empirical validation.

The Psychiatric Evaluation

If this degree of psychopathology among those referred for transplantation is representative, it is understandable that psychiatric assessment is thought to be an important part of the candidate's initial evaluation.

There are at least five putative objectives in such an assessment: (1) the identification of personal strengths and weaknesses that may shape the individual's psychological response to transplantation, (2) the accurate recognition of relative psychiatric contraindications to transplantation, (3) the development of baseline data to formulate plans for specific interventions should they be needed later, (4) the development of therapeutic rapport, and (5) the education of the patient about what to expect regarding possible psychological and psychiatric problems. The overriding goal is to estimate and influence factors that affect treatment compliance and overall outcome.

Also during this process, the potential candidate is prompted to: (1) consider his motives and attitudes regarding transplantation, (2) confront the idea that it is a psychologically potent process, (3) review the effectiveness of his coping styles, and (4) establish a mental set in which he is prepared to work on maladaptive emotional or behavioral symptoms if it becomes necessary.

The psychiatric evaluation should include components from a basic, complete psychiatric evaluation: chief complaints, history of current illness, medications and allergies, habits (tobacco, alcohol, illicit drugs), criminal or antisocial history, past medical history, past psychiatric history, family history (including psychiatric disorders), past personal history (including development, education, relationships, and occupations), psychiatric review of symptoms (from major DSM-III categories), and mental status examination. Other topics that are especially important for the transplant candidate include: (1) history of compliance with medical treatment, (2) behavioral history of hospitalizations, (3) quality of relationships with doctors and nurses, (4) attitudes and knowledge about illness and medications, and (5) major coping strategies for anxiety and demoralization.

A focused evaluation of the patient's spouse or significant other is also important. The spouse often can expand and corroborate the candidate's history and give important clues about issues that may have been overlooked or concealed. He will be the designated provider of emotional support, help, and advocacy; in the event of incapacity this may also be the person making decisions for the patient. If the spouse is unstable, unreliable, or overwhelmed, these kinds of expectations may not be realistic and other individuals would need to be identified to help.

The Psychiatric Interview

Several points about the psychiatric interview deserve emphasis. It is useful to begin with a statement of the purpose of the interview, its scope, and its length. The patient may hold the notion that the psychiatrist's purpose is to uncover a flaw that will invalidate transplant candidacy. Such an erroneous belief obviously would produce anxiety and reticence, and should be corrected early. On the other hand, the patient must understand that the psychiatrist might counsel against transplantation in some circumstances. But there is no veto power. In most cases these decisions are made in a multidisciplinary context in which psychiatric impressions are only a part of the information reviewed by a group in arriving at a decision.

With introductory material out of the way, one might begin with either a brief history of the cardiac illness or focus on the topic of transplantation itself. A chronologic overview of the patient's illness is nearly rote for him by this time, tends to put the patient at ease, and immediately provides important psychiatric information. As one hears about the duration of illness and the degree of disability and suffering, one learns about the patient's predominant coping strategies.

Reliable knowledge about the patient's use of alcohol, drugs, and tobacco is essential. This should be reviewed thoroughly and matter-of-factly with the patient, beginning with open-ended questions like, "Tell me how you have used alcohol through your life?" The perfunctory, true-false question, "Have you ever had a problem with alcohol?", has an understandably high false-negative risk. Follow with questions that tap into symptoms suggesting dependence, blackouts, traffic violations, divorces, and job loss due to alcohol. Has the patient had treatment, sought treatment, or been counseled to get treatment by professionals or family members or friends?

From the developmental history, how a patient coped with his transition from adolescence to adulthood may suggest the style of response that he is likely to use with major life crises such as transplantation. The patient who managed this transition largely by acting out, abusing alcohol, and embroiling himself in conflicts with authority may repeat this and will need extra surveillance, support, structure, and limit-setting. The individual who demonstrated great ambivalence about separating from the family and taking on an independent role in society may later vacillate when it is time to separate from a symbiotic hospital setting after transplantation. Similarly, a person's experience with marriage and close relationships provides clues about his capacity to form and maintain important interpersonal relationships. The middle-aged patient who has never established a close relationship is likely to have a difficult time negotiating the close relationships necessary during transplantation and may need extra involvement with the program psychiatrist or social worker.

Family psychiatric history is important for two reasons. First, it may help confirm impressions about possible prior psychiatric episodes of the candidate. Knowing that a patient with a likely history of several depressive episodes also has a strong family history of affective disorder will help signal the team to be especially watchful for a precipitated depression. Second, a patient with a strong family history of alcoholism or sedative/hypnotic dependence may biologically be at increased risk to develop similar dependence; this will prompt particular caution about the use of benzodiazepines.

A baseline mental status examination must be performed. It should include assessments of general observations, speech, thought, mood, affect, and cognition—problems with diagnostic accuracy notwithstanding.[28] Inquiries should be made about suicidal or homicidal thought, both current and past. The patient should be specifically asked whether he has had hallucinations, delusions, or other symptoms of thought disorder. Positive responses to these questions may suggest a major mental illness but more commonly suggest an episode of significant delirium or organicity associated with either cardiac medications or episodes of cardiac decompensation.

Compliance with medical treatment is closely related to one's attitudes about the illness and its treatment.[29,30] It is important to review carefully the depth and breadth of the patient's knowledge about his heart disease and about its treatment. Whereas the level of sophistication may vary with the patient's prior experience, intelligence, and education level, it would be worrisome if an individual had only the most concrete and naive perception of his illness, was not aware of the name or general purpose of any of his medications, and grossly minimized the extent of his heart disease. Without successful remediation of these lapses in knowledge, the risk of noncompliance is probably substantial.

Psychological Testing

Several reports have mentioned a range of psychological and neuropsychological tests in the evaluation of heart transplant candidates,[14,31] but published findings have not yet appeared. A major question is how to use these data if they are collected. Fundamentally, a conflict arises between how much data are needed to make clinical decisions and how much those data cost in terms of time, effort, and money. At present it appears that routine testing is a research tool. However, selected clinical dilemmas can be greatly clarified by focused neuropsychological consultations. For instance, when organic syndromes are considered, testing can help confirm and quantify even the most subtle deficits.

Additional Testing

Neuropsychiatric complications of heart failure, valvular heart disease, cardiomyopathy, and atherosclerosis are likely to be overrepresented in heart transplant candidates.[32] Brain imaging with computed tomography or magnetic resonance imaging can uncover structural etiologies of some psychiatric presentations. This may help in judging whether a mental syndrome is likely to reverse with transplantation. In selected cases, for instance deciding about whether a psychiatric syndrome is organic or function in order to decide on pharmacologic treatment, an electroencephalogram may be helpful.[33]

Psychiatric Exclusion Criteria

There are no universal psychiatric or psychosocial exclusions to transplantation, even though most centers view as relative contraindications one or more of the following: history of noncompliance, inadequate support systems, ambivalence, psychological denial, psychosis, depression, suicidal behavior, schizophrenia, mental retardation, alcohol or substance abuse, and antisocial personality disorder. Still, the fundamental questions are these: Should otherwise suitable candidates for transplantation ever be denied the opportunity to make use of a successful transplant on the basis of psychiatric or psychosocial criteria? If they should, what are those exact criteria, and on what basis have they been shown to be reliable and valid?

This is a very difficult issue. It is clear that heart transplantation must be rationed, mostly because candidates outnumber donors and because other resources are limited.[13,34] And it seems reasonable to exclude those in whom long-term survival is relatively remote. After all this is the major rationale for excluding otherwise suitable individuals with disseminated malignancy or pulmonary hypertension.

The issue of exclusions on psychiatric grounds largely centers on an estimation of a person's ability to comply with medical management and avoid undue risks to the transplanted organ. Concretely, this requires of the patient compulsive adherence to a medication schedule that frequently produces adverse side effects, commitment to a follow-up system that includes indefinite surveillance and treatment, and active maintenance of general health in a responsible way—no drinking, smoking or "doing drugs". Not everyone can accomplish this.

The problem is that criteria and methods to distinguish prospectively those patients who can comply from those who cannot have not been validated. Understandably, several centers have indicated that they do not generally exclude patients categorically, but in taking this tact they later found troublesome rates of morbidity and mortality as a result of noncompliance.[1,35] Other centers are unclear about the exact criteria they use, but do describe examples of problems that warrant exclusion. Overall, there only appears to be consensus about excluding some candidates with antisocial personality disorder, particularly when this is associated with a pattern of alcohol or substance abuse. For the time being, the most expeditious compromise is probably to accept the practicality of prudent psychiatric/psychosocial exclusions while maintaining a robust scepticism about their precision. Obviously, a major challenge for psychiatrists in heart transplant programs in the future will be to establish better standardized evaluations and demonstrate validity and reliability regarding these issues.

Serious Mental Syndromes in Recipients

Four types of serious psychiatric syndromes are encountered in transplant recipients: delirium, psychosis, mania, and depression.[2] Delirium is characterized by fluctuating level of consciousness and inability to sustain and shift attention appropriately. It is usually marked by significant disorientation, mental confusion, and disorganized delusional thoughts. Psychosis frequently overlaps with delirium but in psychosis, hallucinations, organized delusions, and relative preservation of orientation, cognition, and level of consciousness are usually more prominent. Mania is usually recognized by euphoria, expanded psychomotor energy, grandiosity, and hypersexual behavior; however, some with this reaction appear predominantly irritable, paranoid, and confused. Depression, perhaps the most common syndrome in recipients, is identified by statements or behavior that reflect hopelessness, helplessness, guilt, thoughts of death or suicide, inability to experience pleasure, and vegetative disturbances of appetite, sleep, and physical energy. Correct interpretation of the latter is frequently confounded by the co-existing medical conditions of recently transplanted patients. Although these four syndromes are more likely to appear early in the first few postoperative months, they can occur at any point in the course of the patient's care.

Establishing the exact etiology of any of these four states can be difficult. If an acute medical problem such as hypoxia, hypotension, generalized sepsis, or encephalitis parallels the syndrome, it is generally viewed as organic, particularly if cognition is significantly impaired. Without such medical clues one is usually left to speculate about effects of anesthesia, mechanical perfusion, intercurrent medical problems, corticosteroids, and other medications versus various psychosocial factors. Some support for each of these elements is often present and one frequently settles for a multifactorial explanation. Nonetheless, it is very important to evaluate possible organic etiologies as best one can because neurological complications of transplantation[36,37] may initially present behaviorally. Particularly in the case of delirium, exhaustive attempts to find reversible medical causes should be made.

Delirium

Well trained intensive care nursing staff have little difficulty identifying frank delirium and managing it effectively by repeatedly re-orienting the patient, providing reality testing with simple concrete statements, monitoring and controlling agitated behavior, and minimizing environmental contributions to delirium such as sleep deprivation, ambiguous noises, and isolation. But more subtle mental changes, particularly if they lead to irritability or nastiness, uncooperativeness, or passivity, are sometimes viewed inaccurately as reflections of a personality disorder. An explanation of how the patient's cognitive deficits substantiate the organic basis of these problems can usually clarify this.

The central treatment of delirium is to remove all possible inciting causes and to employ conservative symptomatic management.[38] The patient's behavior must be supervised carefully. Depending on the setting, consideration should be given to one-to-one nursing, physical restraints, and the availability of back-up support. The addition of psychotropic drugs will not reverse delirium, although it may be necessary to manage dangerous or disruptive behavior. Low-dose, high potency antipsychotic agents are most frequently used.[38] Doses should be titrated against specific behavioral signs (e.g., haloperidol 2 mg intramuscularly q 4h, while the patient is agitated or hostile; hold the dose if patient appears sedated). As needed, or "PRN," doses in delirium lasting several days often lead to erratic fluctuations in total daily dose and require that the patient's behavior deteriorate in order to prompt a predictably needed dose. Low potency antipsychotic agents such as chlorpromazine are best avoided because their anticholinergic effects may exacerbate the delirium rather than ameliorate it. Benzodiazepines can be used as an adjunct for additional sedation in some patients but are also best avoided because they may worsen and prolong the delirium. Medical, surgical, and nursing staff need to be reminded that patients who are delirious may have incredibly disordered perceptions and ideas as part of their delirium and can act out impulsively in a dangerous way with little warning.

For patients recovering from delirium, it is important to recognize that they can appear largely personality disordered with impatient, demanding, erratic, inconsiderate or rude behavior as mental improvement progresses from frank delirium to normality. Nonetheless, limits need to be set on this transitional behavior and the medical and nursing staff may need, at times paradoxically, frequent support to set these limits.

Psychosis

The initial treatment of psychosis in this setting is similar to that of delirium but the amount of nursing supervision, environmental restraints, and medication dosages must be tailored to the syndrome. For instance, the patient with paranoid ideas requires consistent and guarded observation from a distance. He may respond aggressively to attempts at control or restraint, and his treatment may thus require more emphasis on pharmacologic controls. Patients with paranoia who also appear to have a fearful or tormented affect are at considerable risk to act out in dangerous ways, and the medical and nursing staff should be repeatedly cautioned about this. Obviously, if feasible, this circumstance is probably better managed on a psychiatric unit of the hospital.

Mania

Mania is probably most common early after transplantation and is often described as manic or hypomanic because of an exaggerated sense of rejuvenation, health, relief, and optimism. But some patients have alterations in level of consciousness with fluctuations in alertness and other symptoms: hallucinations, paranoia, confusion, and difficulty sustaining and shifting attention. The elation, optimism, and mild psychomotor agitation soon after transplantation is best observed and controlled behaviorally or environmentally if necessary. If the patient becomes overtly psychotic, close supervision is needed and the use of antipsychotic agents should be considered.

One should begin with low doses and titrate against specific behaviors that initially indicated the use of these agents. Since it is always unclear how great the organic component is, the more anticholinergic and lower potency antipsychotic agents such as chlorpromazine or thioridazine again should probably be avoided. Hypomanic patients often require close observation and repeated limit-setting for control of their disruptive and intrusive behavior. However, most transplant recipients with this reaction are directable and cooperative. Because this response is often short-lived, pharmacotherapy is probably best reserved for the most severe or protracted cases.

Depression

One should not be surprised to see the hypomanic state shift to a depressed or dysphoric state during the first postoperative week or two. In part, this may be a psychological response to adjusting to some of the realities of the transplantation and hospitalization and to the fact that not only do many problems remain but there seem to be new problems each day. It is equally likely that corticosteroids or other medical factors are involved. Again, treatment is best delayed until there is a clear trend and major indications that outweigh the risks of initiating specific treatment.

When organic factors are the cause, it is reassuring to the patient to be told that these are the sources of his depressed and nihilistic thoughts, that his outlook and mood are being affected by medical factors or medications, and that this will pass. It is important to tell him that his impressions and attitudes are false. Diversions and support from others to suspend ruminative and negativistic thoughts are essential. Antidepressant agents do not have a place in the initial treatment of acute depressive syndromes that are caused by organic factors, especially if they can be expected to resolve in a matter of days to weeks.

One exception to this is when the manifestations of the depression have life-threatening effects on the patient's ability to participate in his own recovery or rehabilitation. In these situations, electroconvulsive therapy or psychostimulants should be considered. Recent studies of depressed patients too ill to tolerate antidepressants agents and of patients with human immunodeficiency virus (HIV) encephalopathy/depression have shown relatively rapid benefit from treatment with methylphenidate or dextroamphetamine.[39-41] Persistent depressions lasting longer than 2 weeks and without obvious organic causes should probably be viewed as clinical depression to be treated accordingly: major depression with antidepressant agents alone or in combination with psychotherapy.[42]

Drug-Induced Mental Syndromes

Corticosteroids

Steroid-induced psychiatric syndromes are well known.[43-46] The Boston Collaborative Drug Surveillance Program study (BCDSP) of 718 patients receiving corticosteroids reported an incidence of 3%, but it has been found to be as high as 57% among patients with systemic lupus erythematosus (SLE). Steroid dose appears to be the strongest predictor of incidence. In the BCDSP the incidence was 1.3% for those receiving less than 40 mg of prednisone daily, 4.6% for those receiving between 40 mg and 80 mg daily, and 18.4% for those receiving more than 80 mg daily. Increased incidence is also associated with a family history of psychiatric illness and female sex.[47,48] But, there is no evidence for associations with age, prior psychiatric illness, medical illnesses other than SLE, or a prior history of steroid- induced mental changes.

Most reports indicate great variability in the types of steroid-induced syndromes, but reviews tabulate averaged frequencies as mania 31%, depression 40%, toxic psychosis 16%, and other syndromes 13%.[43] Problems generally appear within a few days to 2 to 3 weeks of beginning treatment. However, recent reports on rapid (daily) mood and behavior cycling with alternate-day dosing[49] suggest that for some the effects can be relatively immediate and recurring. As yet there is no evidence that dose has an effect on time of onset. The duration of the condition in those whose dose is not decreased and who do not receive psychotropic agents is unclear, despite reports that the condition can be self-limited.[43]

The pathophysiology of steroid psychosis is unknown; however, since corticosteroids do affect brain neurotransmitter function,[50] this may be a likely mechanism. Recent discussions suggest that serotonergic function may be important in steroid psychosis[43,51] and that lithium, which has effects on serotonin, may be effective prophylactically.[52]

Remission of steroid-induced mental changes is expected within a matter of days upon withdrawal of the drug. However, this is seldom feasible in transplant recipients who are rejecting their grafts. Thus, one uses the lowest steroid dose consistent with suppressing rejection and manages the mental complications with hospital supervision and empiric psychopharmacologic agents such as antipsychotic agents, lithium, or benzodiazepines. Brief medication courses with low dosage often suffice. For instance, in one study utilizing low potency neuroleptics, the average daily dose of chlorpromazine or thioridazine required was 212 mg[48]; an equivalent dose of a high potency antipsychotic agent such as haloperidol would be 5 to 15 mg. Lithium may have unique advantages in preventing steroid psychosis[52]; however; the question of delay in the onset of action, which would determine its usefulness in acute situations, is unreported for this indication.

Cyclosporine and Other Immunosuppressive Agents

Cyclosporine, azathioprine, and other immunosuppressive agents less commonly produce psychiatric syndromes,[53] although neurotoxicity can be catastrophic.[54,55] One review mentions visual hallucinations, confusion, disorientation, paranoia, anxiety, and apathy in various cases anecdotally associated with cyclosporine,[55] and one report attributes a case of mania to cyclosporine.[56] The pan T cell monoclonal antibody OKT3 has also been associated with vivid nightmares, occasionally hallucinations, and rarely acute pyschosis. More commonly these medications are associated with troublesome physical symptoms that indirectly could exacerbate depression and anxiety.[53]

Cardiac Effects of Psychotropic Agents

Several comprehensive reviews of the cardiac effects of psychotropic agents exist[57,58]; however, there are no published studies that demonstrate whether different effects appear among transplant recipients who are treated with psychotropic agents. At present one must extrapolate known psychotropic mechanisms and relationships from anatomically intact individuals[59] while factoring in the likely effects of complete denervation of the transplanted heart. Unfortunately, such estimations are complicated further by potential drug interactions with the many different medications used in the medical management of these patients, particularly immunosuppressive, antihypertensive, and antiarrhythmic agents.

Antidepressant Agents

The important side effects of many antidepressant agents generally stem from their interaction with adrenergic, cholinergic, and histaminic neurotransmitter systems.[59] In particular, it is believed that alpha-adrenergic blockade leads to reduced vascular tone and sluggish orthostatic reflexes, and cardiac compensation for this in the transplant recipient is impeded by sympathetic and vagal denervation of the heart. As a result, orthostatic hypotension can occur and may even necessitate hospitalization and intravenous fluids. Furthermore, milder orthostasis may be involved in a portion of the complaints of cognitive problems and fatigue in some patients. For this reason, tertiary amines such as amitriptyline, imipramine, and doxepin, which have greater affinity for alpha- adrenergic receptors, are likely to produce more problems than their secondary amine derivatives, such as nortriptyline and desipramine.[40] Newer antidepressant agents may have advantages for transplant patients, since in the case of fluoxetine there are no reported alpha-adrenergic blocking properties and few other side effects.[50,60]

The peripheral anticholinergic effects of antidepressant agents (e.g., xerostomia, mydriasis, constipation) in transplant recipients are probably not different from other patients and vagal effects on the heart (tachycardia) would be expected to be absent because of denervation. Whereas sedating anticholinergic and antihistaminic side effects are generally unwanted in recipients, occasional patients welcome these as a soporific. Of more concern is the possibility that anticholinergic activity may have delirium-producing potential,[61] particularly among patients already at substantial risk because of metabolic perturbations, additive effects with other medications, or intercurrent acute illnesses such as infection.

The cardiotoxic potential of tricyclic antidepressant agents is well known,[40] in part because of their frequent use in suicidal overdoses, underscoring their narrow therapeutic index. With appropriate doses and drug level monitoring, this is much less a problem.[40,62] There is little evidence that the experimental findings of depressed inotropy are clinically important.[40] Quinidine-like effects of tricyclic agents may make their use risky in patients with conduction defects, particularly with blocks of greater than first degree.[57] However, for the same reason they may be advantageous in patients with ectopy and tachyarrhythmias.[51]

Antipsychotic Agents

Many antipsychotic agents also have anticholinergic and alpha- adrenergic blocking effects,[59] so the same cautions regarding tricyclic agents also apply here. They, too, are associated with a variety of metabolic and electrocardiographic effects on myocardial tissue and can produce myocardial depression and hemodynamically significant arrhythmias.[57] To date, though, no reports have appeared of such effects in transplant recipients, and, except for mechanisms that rely on an innervated heart, cardioactive effects of antipsychotic agents should not differ substantially from those that are well known.[57] Idiosyncratic electrocardiographic catastrophes have been described and appear to be more commonly reported with low potency antipsychotic agents such as chlorpromazine or thioridazine.[57] Thus, thiothixine (Navane), molindone (Moban), and haloperidol (Haldol) may be safer, but convincing comparative studies are unavailable. It is remarkable that given the many theoretical adverse effects of antipsychotic agents, several studies report salutary hemodynamic effects of antipsychotic agents at relatively low doses.[57]

Antipsychotic agents can interact with an array of other medications used in cardiac patients, including sympathomimetics, digoxin, thiazides, antiarrhythmics, quinidine, anticoagulants, anticholinergics, and central nervous system depressants.[57] Thus, the clinician should appraise these effects thoroughly when adding antipsychotic agents to already complex drug combinations. Finally, the clinician using antipsychotic agents must be familiar with the recognition and treatment of (1) common extrapyramidal syndromes associated with antipsychotic agents: acute dystonias, akathisia, parkinsonism, and tardive dyskinesia,[63] and (2) neuroleptic malignant syndrome.[64]

Lithium

Lithium is the preferred treatment of bipolar affective disorder and has been used in a variety of other neuropsychiatric conditions.[65] Its use would need to be considered in recipients with such a history, in addition to its possible use in steroid- induced syndromes. Beyond its more familiar neurological and gastrointestinal side effects, lithium has infrequently been implicated in T-wave changes, conduction abnormalities, and arrhythmias at therapeutic and toxic blood levels.[66] Because of lithium's numerous physiologic actions,[65] the clinician should be circumspect with its prescription in transplant recipients.

Benzodiazepines

Because of their effectiveness and safety,[67-69] benzodiazepines are the preferred antianxiety agent or sedative/hypnotic when these effects are sought. Reports of adverse cardiac effects among heart transplant patients have not been described. Indeed, the prevalence of their use is unreported, despite reports that anxiety is a major problem. Benzodiazepines have little or no cardiovascular toxicity.[57] In addition to their routine use by cardiologists as an amnestic agent in cardioversion, they have been reported to be useful as antiarrhythmics in some refractory patients, and have even been said to have coronary vasodilatory effects.[57] The risks in the transplant recipient include delirium or other organic mental states, altered alertness, disinhibition, paradoxical agitation, and drug dependence and withdrawal phenomena.[69] Thus, even with these preparations the clinician should remain wary.

Conclusion

The adaptive psychological stages of cardiac transplantation illustrate that transplantation is best viewed as a complex, ongoing process in the patient's life, rather than as a static event. Psychiatric disorders can occur at any point during this process and can be recognized using conventional psychiatric approaches. Because of the complex physiology and pharmacology of tranplantation, extra attention and thought are required in the biological treatment of these disorders. There are many unanswered questions about selection/exclusion evaluations and other psychiatric aspects of heart transplantation. Nonetheless, clinical needs among these patients argue for ongoing psychiatric involvement.

References

1. Kuhn WF, Davis MH, Lippman SB. Emotional adjustment to cardiac transplantation. *Gen Hosp Psychiatry*. 1988;10:108–113.
2. Watts D, Freeman AM, McGiffin DG, et al. Psychiatric aspects of cardiac transplantation. *J Heart Transplant*. 1984;3:243–247.

3. Christopherson LK. Cardiac transplantation: a psychological perspective. *Circulation*. 1987;75:57–62.

4. O'Brien VC. Psychological and social aspects of heart transplantation. *J Heart Transplantation*. 1985;4:229–231.

5. Brennan AF, Davis MH, Buchholz DJ, et al. Predictors of quality of life following cardiac transplantation. *Psychosomatics*. 1987;28:566–571.

6. Freeman AM, Foks DG, Sokol RS, et al. Cardiac transplantation: clinical correlates of psychiatric outcome. *Psychosomatics*. 1988;29:47–54.

7. Christopherson LK, Lunde DT. Selection of cardiac transplant recipients and their subsequent psychosocial adjustment. In: Castelnuovo-Tedesco P, ed. *Psychiatric Aspects of Organ Transplantation*. New York, NY: Grune & Stratton; 1971:36–45.

8. Chang VP, Spratt PM, Baron D. Selection of patients for cardiac transplantation. *Med J Aust*. 1985;142:288–289.

9. Mai FM, McKenzie FN, Kostuk WJ. Psychiatric aspects of heart transplantation: preoperative evaluation and postoperative sequelae. *Br Med J*. 1986;292:311–313.

10. Merrikin KJ, Overcast TD. Patient selection for heart transplantation: when is a discriminating choice discrimination? *J Health Polit Policy Law*. 1985;10:7–32.

11. Myers B, Kuhn WF. Informed consent issues in the cardiac transplantation evaluation. *Bull Am Acad Psychiatry Law*. 1988;16:59–66.

12. Marsden C. Ethical issues in a heart transplant program. *Heart Lung*. 1985;14:495–498.

13. Annas GJ. The prostitute, the playboy and the poet: rationing schemes for organ transplantation. *Am J Public Health*. 1985;75:187–189.

14. Frierson RL, Lippmann SB. Heart transplant candidates rejected on psychiatric indications. *Psychosomatics*. 1987;28:347–355.

15. Midelfort J. The psychosocial aspects of heart transplantation. In: Myerowitz PD, ed. *Heart Transplantation*. Mount Kisco, NY: Futura Publishing Co; 1987:283–307.

16. Caine N, O'Brien V. Quality of life and psychological aspects of heart transplantation. In: Wallwork J, ed. *Heart and Heart-Lung Transplantation*. Philadelphia, Penn: WB Saunders Co; 1989:389–422.

17. Slaby AE, Glicksman AS. *Adapting to Life-Threatening Illness*. New York, NY: Praeger; 1985.

18. Nash ES. Psychiatric aspects. In: Cooper DKC, Lanza RP, eds. *Heart Transplantation*. Lancaster, Penn: MTP Press; 1984:235–242.

19. Levenson JL, Olbrisch ME. Shortage of donor organs and long waits. *Psychosomatics*. 1987;28(3):399–403.

20. Evans RW, Manninen DL, Maier A, et al. The quality of life of kidney and heart transplant recipients. *Transplant Proc*. 1985;17:1579–1582.

21. Lough ME, Lindsey AM, Shinn JA, et al. Life satisfaction following heart transplantation. *J Heart Transplant*. 1985;4:446–449.

22. Harvison A, Jones BM, McBride M, et al. Rehabilitation after heart transplantation: the Australian experience. *J Heart Transplant*. 1988;7:337–341.

23. Meister ND, McAleer MJ, Meister JS, et al. Returning to work after heart transplantation. *J Heart Transplant*. 1986;5:154–161.

24. Christopherson LK, Griepp RB, Stinson EB. Rehabilitation after cardiac transplantation. *JAMA*. 1976;236:2082–2084.
25. Kuhn WF, Myers B, Brennan AF, et al. Psychopathology in heart transplant candidates. *J Heart Transplant*. 1988;7:223–226.
26. Mai FM. Graft and donor denial in heart transplant recipients. *Am J Psychiatry*. 1986;143:1159–1161.
27. Kay J, Bienenfeld D. Psychiatric qualifiers for heart transplant candidates. *Psychosomatics*. 1988;29:143–144.
28. Keller MB, Manschreck TC. The bedside mental status examination: reliability and validity. *Compr Psychiatry*. 1981;22:500–511.
29. Eraker SA, Kirscht JP, Becker MH. Understanding and improving patient compliance. *Ann Intern Med*. 1984;100:258–268.
30. Stoudemire A, Thompsons TL. Medication noncompliance: systematic approaches to evaluation and intervention. *Gen Hosp Psychiatry*. 1983;5:233–239.
31. McAleer MJ, Copeland J, Fuller J, et al. Psychological aspects of heart transplantation. *J Heart Transplant*. 1985;4:232–233.
32. Reich P, Regestein QR, Murawski BJ, et al. Unrecognized organic mental disorders in survivors of cardiac arrest. *Am J Psychiatry*. 1983;140:1194–1197.
33. Hughes JR. *EEG in Clinical Practice*. Boston: Butterworths; 1982.
34. Evans RW, Manninen DL, Garrison LP, et al. Donor availability as the primary determinant of the future of heart transplantation. *JAMA*. 1986;255:1892–1898.
35. Cooper DKC, Lanza RP, Barnard CN. Noncompliance in heart transplant recipients: the Cape Town experience. *J Heart Transplant*. 1984;33:248–253.
36. Britt RH, Enzmann DR, Remington JS. Intracranial infection in cardiac transplant recipients. *Ann Neurol*. 1981;9:107–119.
37. Hotson JR, Pedley TA. The neurological complications of cardiac transplantation. *Brain*. 1976;99:673–694.
38. Lipowski ZJ. Delirium in the elderly patient. *N Engl J Med*. 1989;320:578–582.
39. Kaufmann MW, Cassem N, Murray G, et al. The use of methylphenidate in depressed patients after cardiac surgery. *J Clin Psychiatry*. 1984;45:82–84.
40. Fernandez F, Adams F, Levy JK, et al. Cognitive impairment due to AIDS-related complex and its response to psychostimulants. *Psychosomatics*. 1988;29:38–46.
41. Chiarello RJ, Cole JO. The use of psychostimulants in general psychiatry. *Arch Gen Psychiatry*. 1987;44:286–295.
42. Paykal ES, ed. *Handbook of Affective Disorder*. New York, NY: Guilford Press; 1982.
43. Ling MHM, Perry PJ, Tsuang MT. Side effects of corticosteroid therapy: psychiatric aspects. *Arch Gen Psychiatry*. 1981;38:471–477.
44. The Boston Collaborative Drug Surveillance Program. Acute adverse reactions to prednisone in relation to dosage. *Clin Pharmacol Ther*. 1972;13:694–698.
45. Marx FW, Barker WF. Surgical results in patients with ulcerative colitis treated with and without corticosteroids. *Am J Surg*. 1967;113:157–164.
46. Cade R, Spooner G, Schlein E, et al. Comparison of azathioprine, prednisone and heparin alone or combined in treated lupus nephritis. *Nephron*. 1973;10:37–56.
47. Rome HP, Braceland FJ. Psychological response to corticotropin, cortisone and related steroid substances: psychotic reaction types. *JAMA*. 1952;148:27–30.

48. Hall RC, Popkin MK, Stickney SK, et al. Presentation of steroid psychoses. *J Nerv Ment Dis*. 1979;167:229–236.
49. Sharfstein SS, Sack DS, Fauci AS. Relationship between alternate-day corticosteroid therapy and behavioral abnormalities. *JAMA*. 1982;248:2987–2989.
50. Meyer JS. Biochemical effects of corticosteroids on neural tissues. *Physiol Rev*. 1985;65:946–1007.
51. Kaufmann MW, Casadonte PE, Peselow ED. Steroid psychosis: treatment advances. *NY State J Med*. 1981;81:1795–1797.
52. Falk WE, Mahnke MW, Poskanzer DC. Lithium prophylaxis of corticotropin-induced psychosis. *JAMA*. 1979;241:1011–1012.
53. Lough ME, Miller JL, Gamberg P. Self-reported change in physical symptoms from cyclosporine-based therapy to azathioprine-based therapy in heart transplant recipients. *J Heart Transplant*. 1986;5:322–326.
54. Berden JHM, Hoitsma JA, Merx JL, et al. Severe central-nervous-system toxicity associated with cyclosporin. *Lancet*. 1985;1:219–220.
55. Walker RW, Brochstein JA. Neurologic complications of immunosuppressive agents. *Neurol Clin*. 1988;6:261–278.
56. Wamboldt FW, Weiler SJ, Kalin NH. Cyclosporin-associated mania. *Biol Psychiatry*. 1984;19:1161–1162.
57. Risch SC, Groom GP, Janowsky DS. The effects of psychotropic drugs on the cardiovascular system. *J Clin Psychiatry*. 1982;43:5 [Sec. 2],16–31.
58. Cassem N. Cardiovascular effects of antidepressants. *J Clin Psychiatry*. 1982;43:11 [Sec. 2],22–28.
59. Baldessarini RJ. *Chemotherapy in Psychiatry*. Cambridge, Mass: Harvard University Press; 1985.
60. Upward JW, Edwards JG, Goldie A, et al. Comparative effects of fluoxetine and amitriptyline on cardiac function. *Br J Clin Pharmacol*. 1988;26:399–402.
61. Golinger RC, Peet T, Tune LE. Association of elevated plasma anticholinergic activity with delirium in surgical patients. *Am J Psychiatry*. 1987;144:1218–1220.
62. Smith RC, Chojnacki M, Hu R, et al. Cardiovascular effects of therapeutic doses of tricyclic antidepressants: importance of blood level monitoring. *J Clin Psychiatry*. 1980;41:12 [Sec. 2], 57–63.
63. Ayd FJ. A survey of drug-induced extrapyramidal reactions. *JAMA*. 1961;175:1054–1060.
64. Levenson JL. Neuroleptic malignant syndrome. *Am J Psychiatry*. 1985;142:1137–1145.
65. Jefferson JW, Greist JH, Ackerman DL. *Lithium Encyclopedia for Clinical Practice*. Washington, DC: American Psychiatric Press; 1983.
66. Mitchell JE, MacKenzie TB. Cardiac effects of lithium therapy in man: a review. *J Clin Psychiatry*. 1982;43:47–51.
67. Dietch J. The nature and entent of benzodiazepine abuse: an overview of recent literature. *Hosp Community Psychiatry*. 1983;34:1139–1145.
68. Greenblatt DJ, Shader RI, Abernethy DR. Drug therapy: current status of benzodiazepines. *N Engl J Med*. 1983;309:354–358,410–416.
69. Lader M, Petursson H. Rational use of anxiolytic/sedative drugs. *Drugs*. 1983;25:514–528.

Appendices

I
Pre- and Postoperative Transplant Orders

The Oregon Health Sciences University
Hospital and Clinics
PHYSICIANS' ORDERS
USE BALLPOINT PEN ONLY. PRESS FIRMLY.

DATE: Mo | Day | Year | Hour

PATIENT DRUG ALLERGIES:

PRE-OPERATIVE ORDERS FOR CARDIAC TRANSPLANT RECIPIENTS

WHEN RECIPIENT ARRIVES ON UNIT (OR FLOOR)

1) Vital signs STAT and q 4 hrs; weight (bed scale) STAT; Old record to floor ASAP.
2) Diet: ____________
   Fluid limit: ____________
3) NPO after _____ except for medications ordered henceforth.
4) Activity ____________
5) STAT PA and lateral chest film in x-ray if possible, otherwise portable film.
6) CBC with 3 part differential, platelet count, electrolytes, PT, PTT, UA, ABG's, -ALL STAT. Routine SMAC. Serum CMV titer.
7) Heart transplant T cell subset count (draw one 5cc purple top tube and one 10cc red top tube). Place 5cc purple top tube on rocker on 7C and call the transplant lab at ×8394 for pickup. If after hours, call in a.m.
8) Type and crossmatch for 6 units packed cells, 4 units FFP. Packed cells must be CMV sero-negative.
9) _____ units platelets (must be CMV sero-negative).
10) Culture throat, sputum (induced if necessary), and urine.

Signature: ____________ M.D.

Location / Room No.

USE BALLPOINT PEN ONLY!

3.99-35

The Oregon Health Sciences University
Hospital and Clinics
PHYSICIANS' ORDERS
USE BALLPOINT PEN ONLY. PRESS FIRMLY.

DATE				PATIENT DRUG ALLERGIES:
Mo	Day	Year	Hour	

				11) Consent forms for heart transplant operation and multiple
				cardiac biopsies to be signed.
				12) Oxygen via _____ at _____L/min.
				13) When final approval given:
				a) Hibiclens shower.
				b) Surgical prep neck to knees, bedline to bedline. Scrub
				entire body with Hibiclens for 10 minutes following
				prep.
				14) After shower insert heparin lock (16 gauge).
				15) Send with patient to OR:
				a) Cefamandole (Mandol) 1 gm vial.
				b) Methylprednisolone 500mg.
				16) Cyclosporin _____mgm po at _____am/pm. Mix
				cyclosporin with 30cc chocolate milk (use glass container),
				have patient drink, rinse container with another 10cc
				chocolate milk and have patient drink that also.
				17) Methylprednisolone 500mg i.v. on call to OR.
				18) Azathioprine _____ mg. i.v. on call to OR.
				19) Cefamandole (Mandol) 1 gm IM or IV on call to OR.
				20) Call results of CBC, electrolytes, platelets, PT, PTT
				to Dr. _____.
				21) If PT ratio > 1.3 give _____ Aquamephyton IM.
				22) NOTIFY ANESTHESIOLOGY THAT RIGHT NECK OR SUB-
				CLAVIAN VEINS MUST NOT BE USED FOR IV LINES.
				23) Allergies:
				Signature:_____M.D.

Location Room No Location Room No Location Room No Location Room No

USE BALLPOINT PEN ONLY!

3.99-35A

The Oregon Health Sciences University
Hospital and Clinics
PHYSICIANS' ORDERS
USE BALLPOINT PEN ONLY. PRESS FIRMLY.

DATE				PATIENT DRUG ALLERGIES:
Mo	Day	Year	Hour	

CARDIAC TRANSPLANTATION

IMMEDIATE POST-OPERATIVE ORDERS

I.   NURSING ORDERS

1) Admit to Cardiac Transplant Unit. Bedrest. ECG monitor.

   Isolation procedure: mask and gloves until all tubes out,

   mask and good hand washing thereafter.

2) V.S. including CVP every 30 minutes and prn until stable,

   then q h and prn.

3) Monitor, notify H.O. FOR:

   a) Systolic BP > _____ or less than _____ mmHg

   b) CVP > _____ or less than _____ mmHg

   c) Temp. > 37.5 degrees C. PO

   d) HR > _____ or less than _____ beats/min

   e) Chest drainage > 250cc/hr

   f) pH > 7.55 or less than 7.35; pCO2 > 40 or less than

      30; p02 > 200 or less than 80.

   g) Serum K + > 5.2 or less than 3.5meq/L

   h) HCT less than 30.

   i) Urine output less than 30cc/hr for 2 consecutive hrs.

   j) Results of first K +

   k) WBC less than 5,000.

4) NPO—Nasogastric tube to low continuous suction.

   Irrigate with NS or change position to keep open.

5) Mediastinal tubes to water seal and suction at 20 cm H2O.

6) Pleural tubes to water seal and suction at 15 cm H2O.

   Signature:_____ M.D.

(Side column labels: Location, Room No.)

USE BALLPOINT PEN ONLY!   **3.**99-36

The Oregon Health Sciences University
Hospital and Clinics
PHYSICIANS' ORDERS
USE BALLPOINT PEN ONLY. PRESS FIRMLY.

DATE				PATIENT DRUG ALLERGIES:
Mo	Day	Year	Hour	

7) Replace chest tube drainage cc for cc with _____ (during the first 24 hr). Blood balance to start at zero, may go + _____ cc. All whole blood packed red blood cells and platelets must be CMV sero-negative. USE CELL SAVER BLOOD FIRST.

8) Foley catheter to gravity drainage. Hourly outputs. Urine specific gravity every 4 hours. Clean meatus with Iodophor swab q shift.

9) Pacemakers:

Atrial _____ @ _____ / min, _____ ma.

Ventricular demand _____ @ _____ /min, _____ ma.

10) Intake and output every one hour.

11) IV's

a) D5W at _____ /hr.

b) Peripheral IV heparin lock. Flush with 2cc heparin flush q 4h (10 units/ml).

c) Keep arterial line patent with heparinized normal saline (1 unit Heparin/ml).

12) Change dressings on all lines, pacemaker wires and tube puncture sites and apply Betadine ointment daily and pm.

13) Rhythm strip q shift and pm.

14) Turn patient side to side q 2 hr.

Signature:_____ M.D.

(side column labels: Location / Room No. repeated)

USE BALLPOINT PEN ONLY!

3.99-36A

The Oregon Health Sciences University
Hospital and Clinics
PHYSICIANS' ORDERS

DATE				PATIENT DRUG ALLERGIES
Mo	Day	Year	Hour	

II. RESPIRATORY

1) Ventilator Mode-IMV

F102 _____

Vt-13cc/kg

Rate-12/min

2) Tracheal suctioning prn-Hyperoxygenate with 100 %

oxygen. May instill 5-10cc sterile NSA prn.

III. MEDICATIONS

1) Morphine Sulfate _____ mgm IV push 1-2 hours prn pain.

2) Cefamandole (Mandol) _____ gm, IV q hrs x 9

3) Furosemide (Lasix) _____ mgm IV q _____ hrs

4) Immunosuppressive therapy

a) Methylprednisolone _____ mgm IV q 12 hrs x 2 doses

b) Azathioprine _____ mg/d IV (hold and notify H.O. if

WBC less than 5,000.)

c) Cyclosporine _____ mgm via NG and clamp x 2 hrs

9 a.m. and 6 p.m. First dose at _____.

Dilute with 30 cc liquid. Rinse container with 10cc

liquid and give also.

d) Mannitol 12.5 gm IV bid with Cyclosporine dose.

5) Ranitidine 50 mg IV bid.

Signature _____ MD

Location *Room No.*

3.99-36B

The Oregon Health Sciences University
Hospital and Clinics
PHYSICIANS' ORDERS

DATE				PATIENT DRUG ALLERGIES		
Mo	Day	Year	Hour			

6). Isoproterenol (5 mgm in 250cc D5W = 20 mcgm/ml) to keep pulse

rate > _____ beats/min. but less than _____ beats/min.

7) Dopamine (800 mgm in 250cc D5W = 3200 mcgm/ml) to keep

systolic BP > _____.

8) Nitroprusside (200 mgm in 250cc D5W = 800 mcgm/ml to keep

systolic BP less than _____ mmHg.

9) KCL: Administer maximum of 5, 10, 20 (circle which) mEq/hr to

keep K + between 4.5 and 5.2mEq/L.

10) Xylocaine: for PVC's > 6/min or V-tach. 100 mg IV and call H.O.

11) Acetaminophen (Tylenol) suppository 600 mg q 4 h prn rectal

temp > 38.5 degrees C.

12) Other medications:

IV. LABORATORY

1) Daily CBD with 3 part differential, SMAC, PT, PTT.

2) HCT and electrolytes stat and every 4 hours.

3) ABG's in 30 minutes, then q 4 hours or 20 minutes after

any ventilator change.

4) Serum Ca + + stat.

5) Q.O.D. urine and sputum or tracheal spirate for routine

and fungal culture.

Signature:_____ MD

Location | **Room No.**

3.99-36C

The Oregon Health Sciences University
Hospital and Clinics
PHYSICIANS' ORDERS

	DATE			
Mo	Day	Year	Hour	

PATIENT DRUG ALLERGIES:

Physicians' Orders
SEND TO UNIT DOSE

6)   Portable chest film stat—then at _____

     and _____; then 7a.m. daily.

7)   ECG in a.m., then M-W-F by ECG department.

8)   Blood—keep 2 units packed cells available

     × 36 hrs. All whole blood, packed red cells

     and platelets must be CMV sero-negative. Type

     and hold as necessary.

Location

Room No.

Physicians' Orders
SENT TO UNIT DOSE

9)   Q M-W-F cyclosporine level. NOTE: CYCLO LEVEL

     MUST BE DRAWN 12 HOURS AFTER THE PREVIOUS DOSE.

_____M.D.

Location

Room No.

Physicians' Orders
SEND TO UNIT DOSE

Location

Room No.

Physicians' Orders
SEND TO UNIT DOSE

Location

Room No.

UNIT DOSE COPY

The Oregon Health Sciences University
Hospital and Clinics
PHYSICIANS' ORDERS

DATE				PATIENT DRUG ALLERGIES
Mo	Day	Year	Hour	

CARDIAC TRANSPLANTATION

POST EXTUBATION ORDERS

I. NURSING CARE ORDERS

1) VS including CVP Q 1 hr. Rectal/oral temp q 2 hrs. ECG monitor.

2) Isolation procedure: Mask and gloves untiol all tubes out;

   mask and good handwashing thereafter.

3) Notify House Officer for:

   a) Systolic pressure > _____ or less than _____ mmHg.

   b) Temp > 37 degrees C. oral.a

   C) HR > _____ or less than _____ beats/minute.

   d) Serum K + > 5.2 or less than 3.5 meq/L.

4) Dangle legs today; out of bed as tolerated in chair.

5) Clear liquid diet, advance to 2 gram Nat/low cholesterol diet

   as tol., with these additional restrictions:

   Total IV/po fluid limit _____ cc/24 hrs.

6) I & O q h.

7) Weigh when chest tube out; then daily at 7 a.m.

Location · Room No. · Location · Room No. · Location · Room No. · Location · Room No.

3.99-37

The Oregon Health Sciences University
Hospital and Clinics
PHYSICIANS' ORDERS

DATE				PATIENT DRUG ALLERGIES
Mo	Day	Year	Hour	

8. Pulmonary:

   a) Oxygen via _____ at _____ L/min.

   b) Incentive spirometer x 10 min. q 2H and prn.

   c) Chest P.T. q 4 hours and prn.

9) Guaiac all stools.

10) IVs

   a) D5W at _____ /hr.

   b) Peripheral IV heparin lock. Flush with 2cc heparin flush

      q 4h (10 units heparin/ml).

   c) Keep arterial line patent with heparinized normal saline

      (1 unit Heparin/ml).

11) Change dressings on all lines, pacemaker wires and tube

   puncture sites and apply Betadine ointment daily and prn.

12) Pacemakers:

   Atrial _____ @ _____ /min, _____ ma.

   Ventricular demand _____ @ _____ /min, _____ ma.

13) Consult Physical Therapy.

II. MEDICATIONS

1) Cefamandol _____ q _____ . Give 2 doses after chest

   tube removal then discontinue.

2) Furosemide (Lasix) _____ mgm IV/po every _____ .

3) Morphine Sulfate _____ mgm IV push every 4-5 hours

   prn pain.

Signature _____ MD

Location

Room No.

3.99-37A

The Oregon Health Sciences University
Hospital and Clinics
PHYSICIANS' ORDERS

DATE				PATIENT DRUG ALLERGIES
Mo	Day	Year	Hour	

4) Isoproteronol (5mgm in 250cc D5W = 20µgm/ml) to keep pulse rate

   > _____ beats/min. but less than _____ beats/min.

5) Nitroprusside (200mgm in 250cc D5W = 800µgm/ml

   to keep systolic BP less than _____ mmHg.

6) Dopamine (800mgm in 250cc D5W = 3200µgm/ml

   systolic BP > _____.

7) Oral medications to be started on the evening of the 1st POD

   a) Cyclosporine ————— mg PO or per NG 9am & 6pm.

      Dilute with 30cc room temperature liquid, drink, rinse container with

      10cc liquid and drink also. Chocolate milk is recommended.

   b) Mannitol _____ gm IV bid with cyclosporine

   c) Azathioprine _____ mgm p.o.q.h.s.

      Notify H.O. and hold for white count less than 5,000.

   d) Prednisone p.o. Dose (mg)

Date	AM	Date	AM

   e) Sucral fate 1 gm po qid.

   f) Ranitidine 150mg po bid.

   g) Antacid _____ 30cc po tid and hs.

   Signature:_____ MD

USE BALLPOINT PEN ONLY!

3.99–37B

Location

Room No.

Location

Room No.

Location

Room No.

Location

Room No.

The Oregon Health Sciences University
Hospital and Clinics
PHYSICIANS' ORDERS
USE BALLPOINT PEN ONLY. PRESS FIRMLY.

DATE				PATIENT DRUG ALLERGIES
Mo	Day	Year	Hour	

h) D.S.S. (Colace) _____ mg po bid

i) Tylenol #3 1–2 PO q 4–6 hrs pain

j) Halcion 0.25mg po qhs prn.

k) Milk of magnesia _____ cc PO qhs prn constipation.

l) Chlortrimazole troche suck and swallow tid and hs.

m) Other medications:

III. LABORATORY

1) Daily SMAC, CBC with three part differential.

2) HCT and electrolytes every _____ hours.

3) ABG's q 8h X 3.

4) Portable CXR post extubation, then bid x one day, then q a.m.

5) ECG q M-W-F.

6) Q M-W-F cyclosporine level. NOTE: CYCLO LEVEL _MUST_

BE DRAWN 12 HOURS AFTER THE PREVIOUS DOSE.

Location
Room No.
Location
Room No.
Location
Room No.
Location
Room No.

Signature:_____ MD

USE BALLPOINT PEN ONLY!

3.99–37C

The Oregon Health Sciences University
Hospital and Clinics
PHYSICIANS' ORDERS
USE BALLPOINT PEN ONLY. PRESS FIRMLY.

DATE				PATIENT DRUG ALLERGIES
Mo	Day	Year	Hour	

CARDIAC TRANSPLANTATION

TRANSFER ORDERS

I. NURSING ORDERS

1) Transfer to_____.

2) Vital signs q 4 hrs.

3) Notify House Officer for:

    a) systolic pressure >_____ or less than_____ mmHg.

    b) Temp >37° C po

    c) HR >_____ or less than _____ beats/minute.

    d) Serum K+ > 5.2 or less than 3.5 mEq/L.

    e) WBC < 5,000.

4) Ambulation: _____.

    May shower and shampoo when dressings off.

5) Isolation precautions: protective mask and wash hands with

    Phisohex or Hibiciens before entering the room. Personnel

    should avoid contact with other infected patients.

6) Diet: 2gm Na+/low cholesterol with these additional

    restrictions: _____.

    All citrus fruit must be peeled. Consultation with registered

    dietician for discharge diet instruction.

7) Fluid limit _____ cc/day.

8) Intake and output.

9) Weight on arrival and q AM.

Signature:_____ MD

Location

Room No.

USE BALLPOINT PEN ONLY!

3.99–38

The Oregon Health Sciences University
Hospital and Clinics
PHYSICIANS' ORDERS
USE BALLPOINT PEN ONLY. PRESS FIRMLY.

DATE				PATIENT DRUG ALLERGIES
Mo	Day	Year	Hour	

10) Guaiac stools qd.

11) Change dressings on all lines, pacemaker wires and tube puncture

sites and apply Betadine ointment daily and prn.

12) Physical therapy as per standard post-cardiac transplant protocol.

13) Chest physiotherapy q 4h when awake for 3 days. Incentive

spirometry for 10 min q 2h when awake.

14) Anti-embolic stockings when out of bed.

II. MEDICATIONS

1) Cyclosporine _____ mgm PO 9am and 6pm. Dilute in 30cc liquid

of patient's choice. Rinse container with additional 10cc liquid and

have patient drink also. Chocolate milk is recommended.

2) Azathioprine _____ mgm PO qhs. Notify H.O. and hold for white

count less than 5000.

3) Prednisone p.o. (Dose to be given in a.m.)

Date	Dose	Date	Dose

4) Antacids 30cc 2 hrs pc and at hs.

5) Furosemide (Lasix) _____ mg PO every _____.

6) Potassium Chloride _____ mEq. PO _____ x

per day.

Signature:_____ MD

Location / Room No. / Location / Room No. / Location / Room No.

USE BALLPOINT PEN ONLY!

3.99–38A

The Oregon Health Sciences University
Hospital and Clinics
PHYSICIANS' ORDERS
USE BALLPOINT PEN ONLY. PRESS FIRMLY.

DATE				PATIENT DRUG ALLERGIES:
Mo	Day	Year	Hour	

PATIENT DRUG ALLERGIES:

7) Colace PO prn.

8) Propoxyphene HCl (Darvon) _____mg PO q4 hrs prn.

9) Milk of Magnesia _____cc PO q hs prn.

10) Halcion 0.25mg po qhs prn sleep.

11) Chlortrimazole troche suck and swallow tid and hs.

12) Sucralfate 1 gm po qid.

13) Ranitidine 150mg po bid.

14) Patient not to receive enemas.

III. LABORATORY

1) Daily SMAC and CBC with 3 part differential through POD 7,

then M-W-F.

2) Q Mon, Wed, Fri cyclosporine level. NOTE: CYCLO LEVEL

MUST BE DRAWN 12 HOURS AFTER THE PREVIOUS

DOSE.

3) PA and lateral chest film in department qd through POD 7 then

MWF.

4) ECG Monday & Thursday.

5) Q Monday: CMV titer (5cc red top), urine and buffy coat

cultures to Diagnostic Virology.

_____ MD

USE BALLPOINT PEN ONLY!

3.99-38B

The Oregon Health Sciences University
Hospital and Clinics
PHYSICIANS' ORDERS
USE BALLPOINT PEN ONLY. PRESS FIRMLY.

DATE				PATIENT DRUG ALLERGIES:
Mo	Day	Year	Hour	

CARDIAC TRANSPLANTATION
DISCHARGE ORDERS

1) Discharge _____ .

2) Medications (dispense one month supply unless otherwise

   indicated). _____

3) D.S.S. (Colace) 100 mg _____ capsule PO _____ .

4) Furosemide (Lasix) _____ mg _____ .

5) Potassium Chloride _____ mEq po _____ .

6) Tylenol 325mgm 1 or 2 PO q 4-6 prn pain.

7) Halcion 0.25mg po qhs prn sleep.

8) Milk of Magnesia _____ cc qhs prn (_____ bottle).

9) Prednisone _____ mgm PO qd. Dispense 5 mgm tabs.

10) Imuran _____ mgm po qhs.

11) Cyclosporine _____ mgm PO bid (9 am–9pm).

12) Chlortrimazole troche suck and swallow tid and h.s.

13) Ranitidine 150mg po bid.

14) Notify transplant coordinator of impending discharge.

_____ M.D.

Location   Room No   Location   Room No   Location   Room No   Location   Room No

USE BALLPOINT PEN ONLY!

3.99-39

II
Pharmacologic Therapy Pre- and Postcardiac Transplantation

TABLE II.1. Pharmacologic therapy in congestive heart failure.

Acute intravenous therapy	Usual dose ranges
Inotropic agents	
Dobutamine	5–10 µg/kg/min
Dopamine	5–15 µg/kg/min
Amrinone	0.75 mg/kg bolus then 5–10 µg/kg/min
Vasodilators	
Sodium nitroprusside	0.5–5 µg/kg/min
Nitroglycerine	5–50 µg/kg/min
Diuretics	
Furosemide	20–100 mg/dose
Bumetanide	1–5 mg/dose
Ethacrinic acid	50–150 mg/dose
Chlorothiazide	500–1000 mg/dose
Chronic oral therapy	
Inotropic agents	
Digoxin	0.125–0.375 mg/dose q 24 hr
Vasodilators	
Captopril	6.25–50 mg/dose q 6–8 hr
Enalapril	2.5–10 mg/dose q 12 hr
Hydralazine	25–100 mg/dose q 6 hr
Isosorbide dinitrate	10–30 mg/dose q 4–6 hr
Diuretics	
Furosemide	20–160 mg/dose q 12–24 hr
Bumetanide	1–5 mg/dose q 12–24 hr
Metolazone	2.5–5 mg/dose q 12–24 hr

TABLE II.2. Maintenance immunosuppression (OHSU[a] protocols).

"Triple therapy"	
Cyclosporine	8 mg/kg loading dose
	2–4 mg/kg/dose q 12 hr[b]
	(IV dose $\frac{1}{3}$ of oral dose)
Methlyprednisolone IV	1 gm intraoperatively
	125 mg × 2 doses q 12 hr
Prednisone postoperatively	1 mg/kg postoperative day 2 followed by rapid taper over 1 week to 0.5 mg/kg, slow taper to 0.1 mg/kg over next 5 months, maintanance dose 5–10 mg/day
Azathioprine	5 mg/kg IV preoperatively
	2 mg/kg/day postoperatively thereafter
Monoclonal antibody OKT3 induction	
Cyclosporine	8 mg/kg loading dose
	2–4 mg/kg/dose q 12 hr beginning on postoperative day 11[b]
OKT3	5 mg IV q day for 14 days starting on postoperative day 0
Methlyprednisolone IV	1 gm intraoperatively
	125 mg × 2 doses q 12 hrs
Prednisone postoperatively	1 mg/kg postoperative day 2 followed by rapid taper over 1 week to 0.5 mg/kg; slow taper to 0.1 mg/kg over next 5 months; maintanance dose 5–10 mg/day
Azathioprine	5 mg/kg IV preoperatively
	2 mg/kg/day postoperatively thereafter

[a]Oregon Health Sciences University.
[b]Dose based on blood cyclosporine levels.

TABLE II.3. Therapy for acute rejection (OHSU[a] protocols).

Low-dose steroids (used for early moderate rejection)	
Prednisone (postoperatively)	3 mg/kg/day for 5 days; rapid taper to maintanance therapy over 2 days
High-dose steroids (used for advanced moderate rejection)	
Prednisone (postoperatively)	5 mg/kg for 5 days; rapid taper to maintanance therapy over 3 days
or	
Methylprednisolone (IV)	1 gm/day for 3 days
OKT3 (used for steroid resistant rejection)	
OKT3	5 mg/day for 10 days (cyclosporine dose reduced by $\frac{1}{2}$ during therapy)
Methotrexate (used for smoldering rejection)	
Methotrexate (postoperatively)	5 mg/day, 2 days/week for 6 weeks, if rejection persists, may repeat 6 week course at 10 mg/day, 2 days/week

[a]Oregon Health Sciences University.

TABLE II.4. Therapy for cyclosporine-induced hypertension.

Arteriolar dilators	
Hydralazine	10–25 mg/dose q 6–8 hr
Minoxidil[a]	2.5–10 mg/dose q 12–24 hr
Angiotensin-converting enzyme inhibitors[b]	
Captopril	6.25–550 mg/dose q 6–8 hr
Enalapril	2.5–10 mg/dose q 12–24 hr
Lisinopril	10–40 mg/dose q 24 hr
Calcium channel blockers[c]	
Nifedipine	10–30 mg/dose q 8 hr
Nifedipine-extended release	30–90 mg/dose q 24 hr
Verapamil	40–120 mg/dose q 8 hr
Verapamil-extended release	240 mg/dose q 12–24 hr
Diltiazem	30–90 mg/dose q 6–8 hr
Diltiazem-extended release	60–120 mg/dose q 12–24 hr
Centrally acting agents	
Methlydopa	250–500 mg/dose q 6–8 hr
Clonidine	0.1–1 mg/dose q 12 hr

[a]Minoxidil should be reserved for hypertension not controlled by less potent therapy. The major side effect is fluid retention and peripheral edema.

[b]Despite usually low renin levels in cyclosporine-induced hypertension, the angrotension-converting enzyme inhibitors do have efficacy in some individuals.

[c]The calcium antagonists verapamil and diltiazem (and nifedipine to lesser amount) inhibit the metabolism of cyclosporine. Levels have to be followed carefully and adjusted accordingly when instituting these agents. Nifidipine is in our experience the most effective antihypertensive in cyclosporine hypertension. However, it is poorly tolerated in most patients, with side effects that include flushing, hypotension, and peripheral edema. The long-acting preparation may be better tolerated.

TABLE II.5. Lipid-lowering agents.

Bile acid bindings[a]	
Colestipol	7.5–15 gm/dose q 12 hr
Cholestyramine	9 gm/dose q 4–24 hr
Lipoprotein metabolism	
Clofibrate	1 gm/dose q 12 hr
Gemfibrozil	600 mg/dose q 12 hr
Probucol	500 mg/dose q 12 hr
Lovastatin[b]	10–20 mg/dose q 12–24 hr
Other	
Niacin	1–2 gm/dose q 8 hr

[a]All bile acid binding agents can also potentially bind cyclosporine, thereby reducing bioavailability. Cyclosporine levels should be monitored frequently.
[b]Cyclosporine has been shown to inhibit the metabolism of lovastatin. This has resulted in extremely high serum levels of lovastatin, which has been reported to cause myocytolysis, myoglobinuria, and renal failure. The starting dose should be 10 mg/day with regular monitoring of serum creatine phosphokinase levels.

Index